A Comprehensive Guide to Robotic Knee Arthroplasty

A Comprehensive Guide to
Robotic Knee Arthroplasty

Editors

Pramod Bhor MBBS MS(Orthopedics)
Fellowship in Arthroplasty
Professor of Orthopedics
Director
Department of Orthopedics and Joint
Replacement Surgery
Robotic Joint Replacement Surgeon
Fortis Hiranandani Hospital, Vashi
Kharghar Medicity Hospital, Kharghar
Navi Mumbai, Maharashtra, India

Sachin Yashwant Kale MBBS MS(Orthopedics)
FCPS D.Ortho Fellowship in Arthroplasty
Past President NMOA, EC Member BOS
Professor and Unit Head
Department of Orthopedics
DY Patil University School of Medicine
Fortis Hiranandani Hospital, Vashi
Apollo Hospital, Belapur
Navi Mumbai, Maharashtra, India

Co-Editors

Sanjay Dhar MBBS MS(Orthopedics)
DNB(Orthopedics)
Professor and Unit Head
Department of Orthopedics
DY Patil University School of Medicine
Navi Mumbai, Maharashtra, India

Sourabh Kulkarni MBBS MS(Orthopedics)
Fellowship in Joint Replacement Surgery
Orthopedic Consultant and Robotic Joint
Replacement Surgeon, Department of Orthopedics
Shreeyash Orthopaedic Trauma and Joint
Replacement Center
Navi Mumbai, Maharashtra, India

Sunil Shetty MBBS MS(Orthopedics) CCCR PGDHHM
Professor and Unit Head
Department of Orthopedics
DY Patil University School of Medicine
Navi Mumbai, Maharashtra, India

Ashish Phadnis MS(Orthopedics) DNB MRCS
FCPS D.Ortho
Director
Jupiter Hospital
Thane, Maharashtra, India

Sawankumar Pawar MBBS DNB(Orthopedics)
MNAMS FIRJR FAJR
Consultant and Robotics Surgeon
Department of Orthopedic and Robotics Surgery
Fortis Hiranandani Hospital, Vashi
Navi Mumbai, Maharashtra, India

Gaurav Kanade MBBS MS(Orthopedics) Fellowship
in Arthroplasty
Associate Professor
Department of Orthopedics
DY Patil University School of Medicine
Navi Mumbai, Maharashtra, India

Ajay Devda MBBS MS(Orthopedics)
Robotic Assisted Joint Replacement Surgeon
Department of Orthopedic
DY Patil Medical College Nerul, Marengo CIMS Hospital
Ahmedabad, Gujarat, India

Foreword
Neeraj Adkar

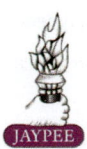

JAYPEE BROTHERS MEDICAL PUBLISHERS
The Health Sciences Publisher
New Delhi | London

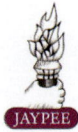

Jaypee Brothers Medical Publishers (P) Ltd

Headquarters
EMCA House, 23/23-B
Ansari Road, Daryaganj
New Delhi 110 002, India
Landline: +91-11-23272143, +91-11-23272703
+91-11-23282021, +91-11-23245672
e-mail: jaypee@jaypeebrothers.com

Overseas Office
JP Medical Ltd.
83, Victoria Street, London
SW1H 0HW (UK)
Phone: +44-20 3170 8910
e-mail: info@jpmedpub.com

Corporate Office
4838/24, Ansari Road, Daryaganj
New Delhi 110 002, India
Phone: +91-11-43574357
Fax: +91-11-43574314
e-mail: jaypee@jaypeebrothers.com

EU GPSR Authorised Representative
Logos Europe, 9 rue Nicolas Poussin
17000, La Rochelle, France
Phone: +33 (0) 6 67 93 73 78
e-mail: contact@logoseurope.eu

Website: www.jaypeebrothers.com
Website: www.jaypeedigital.com

© 2026, Jaypee Brothers Medical Publishers

The views and opinions expressed in this book are solely those of the original contributor(s)/author(s) and do not necessarily represent those of editor(s) or publisher of the book.

All rights reserved. No part of this publication may be reproduced, stored or transmitted in any form or by any means, electronic, mechanical, photocopying, recording or otherwise, without the prior permission in writing of the publishers.

All brand names and product names used in this book are trade names, service marks, trademarks or registered trademarks of their respective owners. The publisher is not associated with any product or vendor mentioned in this book.

Medical knowledge and practice change constantly. This book is designed to provide accurate, authoritative information about the subject matter in question. However, readers are advised to check the most current information available on procedures included and check information from the manufacturer of each product to be administered, to verify the recommended dose, formula, method and duration of administration, adverse effects and contraindications. It is the responsibility of the practitioner to take all appropriate safety precautions. Neither the publisher nor the author(s)/editor(s) assume any liability for any injury and/or damage to persons or property arising from or related to use of material in this book.

This book is sold on the understanding that the publisher is not engaged in providing professional medical services. If such advice or services are required, the services of a competent medical professional should be sought.

Every effort has been made where necessary to contact holders of copyright to obtain permission to reproduce copyright material. If any have been inadvertently overlooked, the publisher will be pleased to make the necessary arrangements at the first opportunity.

Inquiries for bulk sales may be solicited at: jaypee@jaypeebrothers.com

A Comprehensive Guide to Robotic Knee Arthroplasty / Pramod Bhor, Sachin Yashwant Kale

First Edition: **2026**

ISBN: 978-93-7202-289-6

Printed at: Sterling Graphics Pvt. Ltd. India.

Dedication

With deepest gratitude and affection, we dedicate this book to the people and pillars who have made this endeavor possible through their unwavering support, love, and belief in our mission.

To our brilliant editorial team and co-authors

Drs Sanjay Dhar, Ashish Phadnis, Sourabh Kulkarni, Sawankumar Pawar, Sunil Shetty, Gaurav Kanade, Santosh Shetty, Vishal Kumar, Ajay Devda, Kathan Talsania, Gaurav Patel, Sagar Deshpande, Sushant Srivastava, Arvind Vatkar, and Syed Mussadique Ali, and our youngest contributors—Sachiti Sachin Kale and Siddhant Pramod Bhor Your dedication, clinical brilliance, and passion for orthopedics shine through every chapter. This book carries your spirit of teamwork, innovation, and commitment to surgical excellence. We are honored to have collaborated with each one of you.

To our patients

You are our greatest teachers. Each case has taught us far more than any textbook ever could—about resilience, trust, and human spirit. Through your struggles and recoveries, you have shaped us into not only better surgeons but also better people. This book is a tribute to your courage and your trust in us.

To Dr Aditi Bhor, my beloved wife, and our sons, Siddhant and Abhinav

Your boundless love, encouragement, and sacrifices have been the silent strength behind every late-night reading, every long surgery, and every thoughtful moment spent crafting this book. Aditi, your understanding through the unpredictable rhythm of a surgeon's life has been invaluable. Siddhant and Abhinav, your curiosity and smiles remind me daily why I strive to learn, teach, and grow. This journey and this book are as much yours as they are mine.

—Pramod Bhor

To Dr Smruti Kale, my dearest wife, and our daughters, Sachiti and Saanvi

Your quiet strength, unyielding patience, and constant encouragement have helped me push boundaries I never thought I could. Smruti, you are my unwavering anchor, always believing in me even when I doubted myself. Sachiti and Saanvi, your joy and innocence are my daily source of inspiration. Thank you for standing beside me through this demanding yet fulfilling journey.

—Sachin Yashwant Kale

To Fortis Hospital, Vashi—our second home

This institution has not only nurtured our surgical journey but also provided a vibrant academic environment where ideas are born and nurtured. The trust, freedom, and support we have received here have been pivotal in shaping the clinicians and thinkers we are today. Thank you for allowing us to dream big.

With heartfelt gratitude and sincere humility, we dedicate this book to all of you—our families, patients, colleagues, and mentors—who made this labor of love possible.

Pramod Bhor
Sachin Yashwant Kale

Contributors

Ajay Devda MBBS MS(Orthopedics)
Robotic Assisted Joint Replacement
Surgeon, Department of Orthopedics
DY Patil Medical College, Nerul
Marengo CIMS Hospital
Ahmedabad, Gujarat, India

Arvind Vatkar MBBS MS(Orthopedics)
AFIH MCh(Spine Surgery) Advanced Spine
Surgery Fellowship(UK)
Assistant Professor
Department of Orthopedics
MGM Medical College
Navi Mumbai, Maharashtra, India

Ashish Phadnis MS(Orthopedics) DNB
MRCS FCPS D.Ortho
Director
Jupiter Hospital
Thane, Maharashtra, India

Dnyanada Prabodh Kutumbe MBBS
D.Ortho Fellowship in Spine Surgery
Associate Consultant
Department of Orthopedics and
Spine Surgery
Kharghar Medicity Hospital, Kharghar
Acharya Nanesh Hospital, Belapur
Fortis Hiranandani Hospital, Vashi
Navi Mumbai, Maharashtra, India

Gaurav Kanade MBBS MS(Orthopedics)
Fellowship in Arthroplasty
Associate Professor
Department of Orthopedics
DY Patil University School of Medicine
Navi Mumbai, Maharashtra, India

Gaurav Patel MBBS D.Ortho
Arthroplasty Fellow
Department of Orthopedics and Robotic
Joint Replacement
Kharghar Medicity Hospital, Kharghar
Fortis Hiranandani Hospital, Vashi
Navi Mumbai, Maharashtra, India

Kathan Talsania MBBS D.Ortho DNB FIAA
FIAS EFRA
Associate Consultant
Marengo CIMS Hospital
Ahmedabad, Gujarat, India

Neharika Tandon MBBS
PG Student/Resident
Jupiter Hospital
Thane, Maharashtra, India

Pramod Bhor MBBS MS(Orthopedics)
Fellowship in Arthroplasty
Professor of Orthopedics
Director
Department of Orthopedics and
Joint Replacement Surgery
Robotic Joint Replacement Surgeon
Fortis Hiranandani Hospital, Vashi
Kharghar Medicity Hospital, Kharghar
Navi Mumbai, Maharashtra, India

Raj M Sawant MBBS MS(Orthopedics)
DNB(Orthopedics) FIJR
Fellow
Department of Orthopedics
Fortis Hiranandani Hospital, Vashi
Navi Mumbai, Maharashtra, India

Sachin Yashwant Kale MBBS
MS(Orthopedics) FCPS D.Ortho Fellowship in
Arthroplasty
Past President NMOA, EC Member BOS
Professor and Unit Head
Department of Orthopedics
DY Patil University School of Medicine
Fortis Hiranandani Hospital, Vashi
Apollo Hospital, Belapur
Navi Mumbai, Maharashtra, India

Sachiti Sachin Kale MBBS(Third Year)
Student, Lokmanya Tilak Medical College
and Sion Hospital
Mumbai, Maharashtra, India

Contributors

Sagar Deshpande BPT
MPT(Physiotherapy in Neurosciences)
Associate Professor
Department of Neurophysiotherapy
School of Physiotherapy,
DY Patil University
Navi Mumbai, Maharashtra, India

Sanjay Dhar MBBS MS(Orthopedics)
DNB(Orthopedics)
Professor and Unit Head
Department of Orthopedics
DY Patil University School of Medicine
Navi Mumbai, Maharashtra, India

Santosh Shetty MBBS FAGE
MS(Orthopedics) Mch(Orthopedics)
Director and Head
Department of Orthopedics and
Joint Replacement Surgery
Surana Group of Hospitals, Mumbai
CritiCare Asia Group of Hospitals
Fortis, Navi Mumbai
Cumballa Hill Hospital
Maharashtra, India

Sawankumar Pawar MBBS
DNB(Orthopedics) MNAMS FIRJR FAJR
Consultant and Robotics Surgeon
Department of Orthopedics and
Robotics Surgery
Fortis Hiranandani Hospital, Vashi
Navi Mumbai, Maharashtra, India

Shivam Mehra MBBS MS(Orthopedics)
Short-term fellowship in Deformity
Correction and Limb lengthening surgery
(Paley's Institute, Florida) Short-term
Fellowship in Pediatric Upper Limb Deformity
(NCCHD Tokyo, Japan) Deformity Correction
and Limb lengthening, Trauma, Arthroplasty
Consultant
Department of Orthopedics
Mehra Hospital and Research Institute
Lucknow, Uttar Pradesh, India

Siddhant Pramod Bhor MBBS Student
KJ Somaiya Medical College
Mumbai, Maharashtra, India

Sourabh Kulkarni MBBS MS(Orthopedics)
Fellowship in Joint Replacement Surgery
Orthopedic Consultant and Robotic Joint
Replacement Surgeon
Department of Orthopedics
Shreeyash Orthopaedic Trauma and
Joint Replacement Center
Navi Mumbai, Maharashtra, India

Sunil Shetty MBBS MS(Orthopedics)
CCCR PGDHHM
Professor and Unit Head
Department of Orthopedics
DY Patil University School of Medicine
Navi Mumbai, Maharashtra, India

Sushant Srivastava MBBS
MS(Orthopedics)
Assistant Professor
Department of Orthopedics
Mata Gujri Memorial Medical College and
Lions Seva Kendra Hospital
Kishanganj, Bihar, India

Syed Mussadique Ali MBBS
MCh(Orthopedics) DNB(Orthopedics)
MNAMS D.Ortho FIRJR FAJR
Consultant
Department of Orthopedics and
Joint Replacement Surgery
Medicity Hospital Kharghar
Fortis Hiranandani Hospital, Vashi
Navi Mumbai, Maharashtra, India

Vishal Kumar MBBS MS(Orthopedics)
DNB(Orthopedics) FRCS
Adjunct Professor
Department of Orthopedics
Post Graduate Institute of Medical
Education and Research
Chandigarh, India

Foreword

The field of orthopedic surgery is undergoing a profound transformation. As surgeons, engineers, and scientists come together at the intersection of medicine and technology, *robotic-assisted total knee arthroplasty (TKA)* is redefining precision, predictability, and patient outcomes. In this rapidly evolving landscape, a pressing need arises for a consolidated, evidence-based, and practical reference to guide both aspiring and experienced arthroplasty surgeons. "A Comprehensive Guide to Robotic Knee Arthroplasty" fills this critical void.

Edited by *Dr Pramod Bhor* and *Dr Sachin Yashwant Kale*, this book brings together a formidable team of co-editors and contributors—*Drs Sanjay Dhar, Ashish Phadnis, Sourabh Kulkarni, Sunil Shetty, Sawankumar Pawar, Gaurav Kanade, and Ajay Devda*—each of whom brings unique insights and hands-on experience to this futuristic domain. Their combined expertise spans across robotic platforms, alignment philosophies, intraoperative decision-making, and postoperative rehabilitation strategies, making this book both comprehensive and clinically relevant.

This guide begins by addressing the fundamental question—*Why Robotics?*—by examining the inherent challenges of conventional TKR. It then takes readers on a meticulously structured journey, covering the *evolution of robotic technology* and core principles such as *alignment and classification*, and providing detailed discussions on major systems, including *CUVIS, MISSO, MAKO, VELYS, CORI, and ROSA*.

What makes this book truly stand out is its *pragmatic tone and structured clarity*. Each chapter is carefully designed to integrate clinical pearls with technical precision, supported by the authors' vast experience. The chapters on *complication management*, *rehabilitation*, and *real-world advantages* are crucial but often overlooked in clinical practice.

This is more than just a textbook—it is a *blueprint for the future of knee arthroplasty*. As robotic systems continue to evolve and enter operating rooms across the globe, this book will serve as a cornerstone for those who wish to not only adopt but also excel in robotic knee surgery.

I congratulate the editors, co-editors, and all the contributors for producing a timely, well-curated, and immensely valuable work. Whether you are taking your first steps in robotic-assisted surgery or striving to refine your approach, this book is an essential companion on your journey toward *precision orthopedics*.

Neeraj Adkar
Chairman, Managing Director and
Chief Robotic Joint Replacement Surgeon
SaiShree VitaLife Hospital
Pune, Maharashtra, India

Preface

Orthopedic surgery stands at a transformative crossroads, where precision, personalization, and technological innovation are reshaping conventional practices. One of the most significant advancements in recent years is the integration of robotic technology into total knee arthroplasty (TKA). Once considered futuristic, robotic-assisted knee replacement has now become an essential and evolving aspect of modern surgical care, offering improved accuracy, consistency, and patient outcomes.

As orthopedic surgeons who have navigated the transition from traditional to technology-driven arthroplasty, we have experienced firsthand the challenges, questions, excitement, and promise that come with adopting robotic surgery. With this book, "*A Comprehensive Guide to Robotic Knee Arthroplasty*," we aim to bridge the knowledge gap and provide a complete, practical, and unbiased guide for all those navigating this new landscape—be it residents in training, early-career surgeons, or seasoned practitioners.

This book was conceived in response to a genuine need for a single, authoritative resource that not only explains the mechanics of various robotic platforms but also contextualizes their use in real-world clinical scenarios. It is not merely a compilation of theoretical chapters; rather it represents the shared experience of orthopedic surgeons who have collectively performed thousands of robotic knee surgeries. It brings together the knowledge and insights of contributors who are innovators, educators, and front-line clinicians deeply engaged with this technology on a day-to-day basis.

Throughout this book, we have made a conscious effort to keep the content evidence-based, yet clinically oriented and easy to navigate. The chapters begin with the evolution and rationale behind robotic TKA and gradually unfold into detailed discussions on different robotic systems—CUVIS, MISSO, MAKO, VALYS, CORI, ROSA, and more. Each system is examined with a focus on its unique features, operational workflow, indications, benefits, limitations, and clinical outcomes. Comparisons between systems are drawn when relevant to aid in practical decision-making.

We have also given equal importance to often overlooked yet critical topics such as intraoperative challenges, patient selection, learning curves, cost implications, and postoperative protocols, including rehabilitation. These sections are particularly valuable for teams and institutions planning to incorporate robotic TKA into their practice.

A major strength of this book lies in its collaborative spirit. The contributors come from varied practice settings—academic institutes, high-volume centers, and private hospitals—and bring with them diverse perspectives and a shared commitment to patient-centered care. Their willingness to share insights, surgical pearls, and personal learning curves has enriched the value of this resource manifold.

We are deeply grateful to each of them for their dedication, time, and candor. We would also like to express our heartfelt thanks to our families for their unwavering support and patience throughout the process of developing this book. A special mention to our mentors, colleagues, and patients continue to be our guiding lights, inspiring us to innovate, teach, and learn continuously.

In a field as dynamic as robotic knee arthroplasty, knowledge must evolve in tandem with technology. We hope this book will serve not only as a reference but also as a companion—one that instills confidence, encourages critical thinking, and ultimately contributes to better outcomes for patients worldwide.

Let this book be a small step in a larger movement toward precision medicine and surgical excellence.

Pramod Bhor
Sachin Yashwant Kale

Acknowledgments

The journey of creating "*A Comprehensive Guide to Robotic Knee Arthroplasty*" has been deeply enriching—academically, surgically, and personally. This book is the culmination of shared knowledge, collaborative efforts, and unwavering support from many individuals and institutions who have been instrumental in bringing this vision to life.

First and foremost, to our patients
Your trust and resilience continue to inspire us every single day. Every robotic surgery we performed taught us something new—about precision, decision-making, and compassion. This book is, above all, for you.

We express our *deepest gratitude and special mention* to the following *co-editors*, whose leadership, academic integrity, and clinical insight have been instrumental in shaping this work:

Dr Sanjay Dhar
A stalwart in the field of orthopedic surgery and a mentor to many, Dr Dhar's contributions brought academic depth and surgical wisdom to this book. His critical analysis and practical perspectives helped fine-tune key sections, ensuring that the content is both evidence-based and clinically relevant.

Dr Sourabh Kulkarni
Dr Kulkarni's extensive experience in robotic-assisted arthroplasty and his meticulous approach to surgical planning added significant value to the technical portions of this book. His inputs have been crucial in making the content practically applicable and case-oriented.

Dr Sunil Shetty
With his razor-sharp clinical acumen and passion for teaching, Dr Shetty played a pivotal role in curating technically rich and user-friendly chapters. His ability to simplify complex concepts has made this guide an accessible resource for surgeons at every stage of their career.

Dr Ashish Phadnis
A leading robotic joint replacement surgeon at Jupiter Hospital, brings vast experience in robotic knee arthroplasty. He has performed numerous successful robotic-assisted procedures, setting benchmarks in precision and patient outcomes.

As Co-Editor of this book, his insights and clinical expertise have enriched the content, especially in the field of robotic joint replacement.

Dr Sawankumar Pawar

A dynamic and passionate orthopedic surgeon, Dr Pawar brought immense energy and precision to the editorial process. His commitment to accuracy, formatting excellence, and scientific clarity has been vital in shaping this book's final presentation.

Dr Gaurav Kanade

Dr Kanade's expertise in clinical robotics and his innovative mindset contributed richly to the surgical workflow and system comparison sections. His thoughtful suggestions and case-based insights enriched the text and broadened its practical appeal.

Dr Ajay Devda

A rising academician and surgeon, Dr Devda's contributions helped bridge the gap between emerging technologies and day-to-day surgical practice. His collaborative spirit and dedication to detail were truly commendable.

To our exceptional team of contributors

Drs Santosh Shetty, Ashish Phadnis, Sagar Deshpande, Sushant Srivastava, Arvind Vatkar, Syed Mussadique Ali, Vishal Kumar, Kathan Talsania, and Dr Gaurav Patel, and our youngest contributors—Sachiti Sachin Kale and Siddhant Pramod Bhor Thank you for generously sharing your expertise, experiences, and time. Your enthusiasm for robotic technology and commitment to education resonate through every chapter.

A special note of appreciation to Fortis Hospital, Vashi

For providing us with a dynamic academic platform and the freedom to explore, innovate, and evolve. The institutional culture of learning and excellence has played a vital role in shaping both our clinical practice and this publication.

We express our heartfelt gratitude to our families

To Dr Aditi Bhor, Siddhant, and Abhinav.

To Dr Smruti Kale, Sachiti, and Saanvi.

Your patience, sacrifices, and endless encouragement have been the foundation of our ability to pursue this project. Every late night spent in reading, writing, and revising was made possible by your quiet strength and unwavering love.

We extend our sincere thanks to the editorial and production team at Jaypee Brothers Medical Publishers, New Delhi.

For their professionalism, guidance, and seamless execution throughout the publishing process. Jaypee's commitment to medical education and their reputation for academic excellence make them the perfect partner for this project. We are grateful for their belief in the relevance and impact of this work.

Finally, to our mentors, teachers, colleagues, and students.

Thank you for continuously challenging us to learn, adapt, and push boundaries. This book would not have taken shape without the collective wisdom and experience we have absorbed from you over the years.

With deepest respect and appreciation, we acknowledge all those who have supported and inspired us on this journey.

Pramod Bhor
Sachin Yashwant Kale

Contents

1. **Why Robotics? Challenges in Conventional Total Knee Replacement**   1
   Pramod Bhor, Sourabh Kulkarni, Sachin Yashwant Kale, Vishal Kumar, Shivam Mehra

2. **History of Robotics: The Evolution of Robotics in Modern Knee Replacements**   6
   Sawankumar Pawar, Pramod Bhor, Sourabh Kulkarni, Sachin Yashwant Kale, Syed Mussadique Ali, Sachiti Sachin Kale, Siddhant Pramod Bhor, Dnyanada Prabodh Kutumbe

3. **Alignment Strategies in Total Knee Arthroplasty**   12
   Pramod Bhor, Sourabh Kulkarni, Sunil Shetty, Sawankumar Pawar, Syed Mussadique Ali

4. **Components of Robotic System**   23
   Sourabh Kulkarni, Pramod Bhor, Sachin Yashwant Kale, Arvind Vatkar

5. **Classification of Robotic Systems**   30
   Sourabh Kulkarni, Pramod Bhor, Sachin Yashwant Kale, Vishal Kumar

6. **CUVIS Joint Robotic System**   33
   Pramod Bhor, Sawankumar Pawar, Sachin Yashwant Kale, Sourabh Kulkarni, Syed Mussadique Ali, Raj M Sawant

7. **MISSO Robotic System**   51
   Sourabh Kulkarni, Pramod Bhor, Sachin Yashwant Kale

8. **MAKO Robotic System**   66
   Ajay Devda, Kathan Talsania, Sawankumar Pawar, Sachin Yashwant Kale, Pramod Bhor

9. **VELYS Robotic System**   86
   Santosh Shetty, Pramod Bhor, Sachin Yashwant Kale, Sawankumar Pawar, Syed Mussadique Ali, Gaurav Patel, Raj M Sawant

10. **CORI Robotic System**   118
    Ashish Phadnis, Pramod Bhor, Sawankumar Pawar, Gaurav Patel, Sachin Yashwant Kale, Neharika Tandon

11. **ROSA Robotic System**   140
    Gaurav Kanade, Sanjay Dhar, Syed Mussadique Ali

12. **Complication in Robotic Assisted TKA** 177
 Pramod Bhor, Sawankumar Pawar, Sachin Yashwant Kale, Sourabh Kulkarni

13. **Advantages of Robotic Total Knee Replacement** 182
 Pramod Bhor, Sawankumar Pawar, Sachin Yashwant Kale, Sourabh Kulkarni, Shivam Mehra

14. **Rehabilitation in Robotic-guided Knee Arthroplasty** 185
 Sagar Deshpande, Sachin Yashwant Kale, Pramod Bhor, Sushant Srivastava, Sachiti Sachin Kale, Siddhant Pramod Bhor

Suggested Readings 201

Author's Publications 205

Index 207

CHAPTER 1

Why Robotics? Challenges in Conventional Total Knee Replacement

Pramod Bhor, Sourabh Kulkarni, Sachin Yashwant Kale,
Vishal Kumar, Shivam Mehra

INTRODUCTION

Total knee replacement (TKR) and total hip replacement surgeries are one of the most successful surgeries in orthopedics. Conventional joint replacement done by competent surgeons has given amazing results. But humans are defined by inquisitiveness and hunger for progress and precision. The first knee replacement is dated back to 1968. Since 1968, we have done vast improvements in implant design, implant material, polyethylene material, cementing technique, and intraoperative and postoperative management protocols but nothing was done for human-/surgeon-related factors. The success of knee replacement depends on precise alignment, perfect duplication of natural anatomy of a native knee. The gap balancing is also equally important in the success of TKR surgery. Along with this, it is important to standardize and repeat the best results in every case. Achieving this is possible with use of AI and robotics due to various reasons.

ANATOMICAL VARIATIONS

Femoral mechanical-anatomical axis angle (FMMA) as per the studies ranges from 3° to 7° in 75% of the population. Still 25% of the population lies outside this range. So just choosing a femoral zig angle of 5–7° valgus doesn't account for precision.

Intramedullary canal is wide in many patients. in such wide canals intramedullary rod may wobble with 1–3° of variation **(Figs. 1.1A and B)**.

The femoral bow varies amongst individuals and this bow also increases as the age progresses. With severe osteoporotic bowing it has been observed that intramedullary rod abuts the anterior cortex at shorter length. Hence, does not represent the anatomical axis perfectly **(Figs. 1.2A and B)**.

In some cases, it has been observed that FMMA is >10°. But conventional instrumentation sets do not have angle adjustments available.

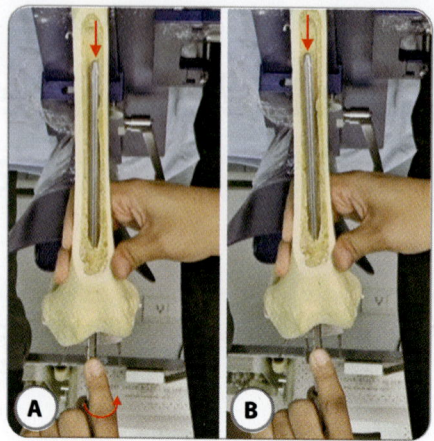

FIGS. 1.1A AND B: Wobble of intramedullary rod.

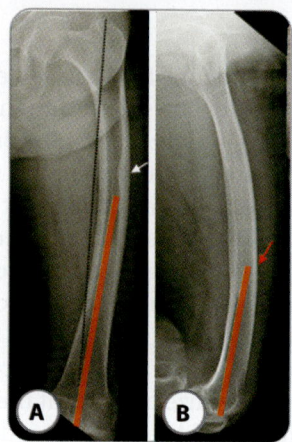

FIGS. 1.2A AND B: Exaggerated femoral bow.

▌MALUNITED FEMUR FRACTURES

In cases of malunited femoral fractures intramedullary canal orientation, diameter and angle are changed. In such cases, the intramedullary canal does not represent the anatomical axis of femur **(Figs. 1.3A and B)**.

▌ERROR OF SAW

It has been observed that there is a possibility of error due to a human hand having various angular forces on a saw blade while cutting through the zig. Also due to friction with the saw blade, zig slots become wider with repeated use, which leads to more play of the saw blade within the slot **(Figs. 1.4A and B)**. As a result, through the same zig slot you can cut a few degrees in varus or valgus and also in different slopes.

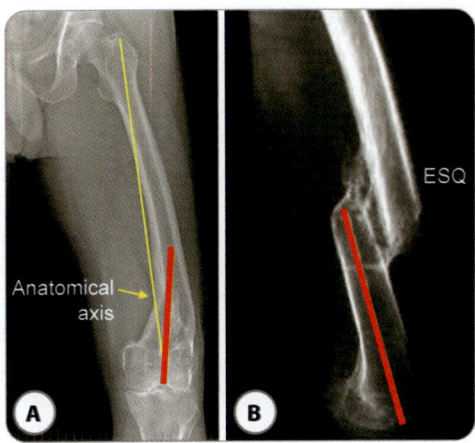

FIGS. 1.3A AND B: Malunited fractures.

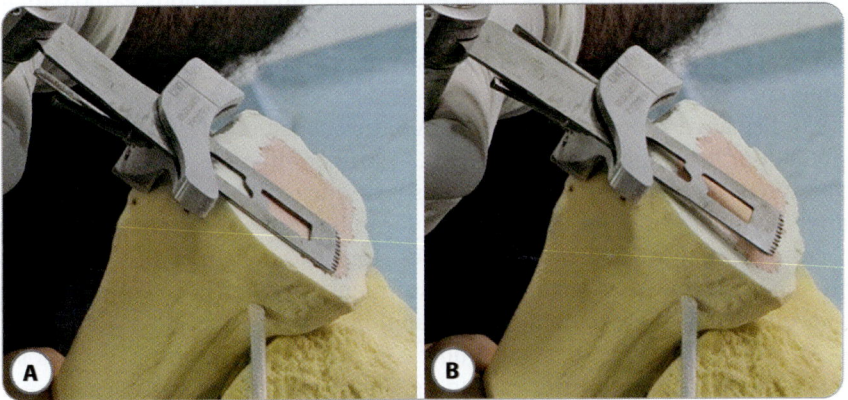

FIGS. 1.4A AND B: Play of saw in zig slot.

ERRORS IN LIGAMENT BALANCING

A submillimeter precision in joint replacement is desirable. This submillimeter difference or variation in medial and lateral gaps is not quantifiable by human eyes. Surgeons can perceive this imbalance but cannot quantify in millimeters. Human eyes also cannot understand angle variations in precise degrees.

In conventional total knee arthroplasty (TKA), we can do gap balancing only after the bone is cut. Intraoperatively to balance the gaps, we might have to do more release leading to insertion of larger poly insert, which retrospectively signifies greater bone loss.

In conventional instrumentation, bone cut can be increased or decreased by 2 mm. Which means for ideal gap balancing if millimeter or submillimeter variation of cut is required, that is not possible.

ALIGNMENT PHILOSOPHY

Recently, there are changes in alignment philosophies for better patient satisfaction and longevity of the implants. It has been changing from mechanical alignment to kinematic alignment. Many surgeons want to practice restricted kinematic alignment where precise limited angle variation is acceptable. In conventional TKA instrumentation being rigid, these angles are difficult to achieve whereas it is easily possible with robotics. Differences between these alignment philosophies and their requisites have been discussed in Chapter 3.

Total knee replacement has long been celebrated as among the most successful procedures in orthopedic practice. With decades of refinement in implant design, material science, and surgical techniques, these operations have drastically improved patients' quality of life. However, despite these advancements, a critical dimension—surgeon- and patient-related variability—has remained relatively unaddressed until the recent advent of artificial intelligence (AI) and robotic-assisted technologies.

The precision required in TKR surgery is immense. Success hinges on accurate anatomical replication, precise limb alignment, and meticulous gap balancing. Yet, these goals are often compromised due to inherent anatomical variations, technical limitations of conventional instruments, and the natural boundaries of human perception and manual dexterity.

Studies have shown that the FMMA varies considerably, and in 25% of the population, it lies outside the typical 3-7° range. In such cases, relying on a fixed valgus angle for distal femoral cuts introduces alignment errors. Similarly, variability in femoral bowing, especially in older or osteoporotic patients, and in cases of malunited femoral fractures, further challenges the reliability of intramedullary guides. Conventional instruments are often not adaptable enough to accommodate these patient-specific anatomical differences.

Moreover, intraoperative execution is prone to human error. Factors such as saw blade play within the cutting jig slots, changes due to repeated use of instruments, and difficulty in achieving submillimeter precision all contribute to inconsistencies in bone cuts and ligament balancing. Surgeons may intuitively perceive imbalance but cannot reliably quantify the exact medial-lateral gap differences or angulation in degrees. This inability to measure and execute with precision can lead to suboptimal outcomes, increased polyethylene wear, instability, or early failure of the prosthesis.

The evolution in alignment philosophies—from mechanical alignment to kinematic and restricted kinematic alignment—further underscores the need for adaptable and patient-specific solutions. Such nuanced approaches, aiming to replicate the native joint mechanics more closely, are exceedingly difficult to implement with conventional tools. Robotic-assisted systems, however, allow for real-time planning, intraoperative customization, and execution with millimetric and subdegree accuracy. This not only helps in achieving perfect alignment but also in preserving soft tissues and minimizing unnecessary bone cuts or releases.

AI and robotics bridge the gap between the surgical plan and its execution. These technologies offer consistent, reproducible, and patient-specific outcomes—mitigating the influence of anatomical variability, reducing intraoperative human error, and allowing alignment philosophies to be accurately implemented. In essence, they enable surgeons to combine their clinical expertise with digital precision.

CONCLUSION

While conventional joint replacement performed by experienced surgeons will continue to yield good results, the integration of AI and robotic technology represents a transformative leap forward. It addresses the long-standing challenge of human and anatomical variability, setting a new standard for consistency, precision, and personalized care in joint arthroplasty. As orthopedic surgery continues to evolve, embracing these technologies is not just an option—it is a necessity for the future of precision joint replacement.

History of Robotics: The Evolution of Robotics in Modern Knee Replacements

*Sawankumar Pawar, Pramod Bhor, Sourabh Kulkarni,
Sachin Yashwant Kale, Syed Mussadique Ali,
Sachiti Sachin Kale, Siddhant Pramod Bhor,
Dnyanada Prabodh Kutumbe*

INTRODUCTION

Total knee arthroplasty (TKA) has evolved from a modest and often unreliable procedure into one of the most successful surgeries in modern orthopedics. Initially overshadowed by hip replacements, early TKAs suffered from poor implant design, limited understanding of biomechanics, and inconsistent results. Over time, advances in implant materials, surgical techniques, and perioperative protocols steadily improved outcomes. The true turning point came with the advent of robotic-assisted TKA, which brought unprecedented accuracy, personalization, and reproducibility. This chapter traces the remarkable journey of TKA—highlighting how continuous innovation, especially through robotics, has transformed knee replacement into a highly precise, patient-centric, and widely successful surgical intervention.

JOURNEY TOTAL KNEE ARTHROPLASTY FROM UNDERPERFORMER TO MOST SUCCESSFUL SURGERY

Total Knee Arthroplasty: The Underperformer

Conventional TKA is one of the safest and most cost-effective orthopedic procedures, with patient satisfaction rates ranging from 75 to 92%. This procedure is a powerful method for pain relief and functional restoration in patients with advanced arthritis after exhausting nonoperative options. Knee replacement surgery, as one currently knows it, started to take shape during the 1960s once hip replacements had unequivocally shown their transformative possibilities for hip arthritis. Hip replacement surgery stimulated an avid interest of knee surgeons in attempting to replicate such results with knee joints. The knee joint by its very nature was more complicated due to intricate biomechanics and load-bearing role. In the early era, there was no uniformity in designs or standards in surgical technique. Even with this limitation apparently all at once many surgeons and engineers gave into this tempting method leading to numbers of failures indicating how we had limited knowledge of knee mechanics, material specifications, and wear patterns.

Total Knee Arthroplasty: The Success

The 1970s and early 1980s were rather exciting times for knee replacement surgery. Improvements in implant design, including modular components and more durable materials, heralded a turning point. Running parallel was the improvement in surgical technique, including better instrumentation and alignment guides, which enhanced the reproducibility and success rates of knee arthroplasty.

It wasn't until the combining of superior surgical techniques and their wide diffusion within the orthopedic community that over time greatly improved the results, increasing the number of knee replacement surgeries.

The methods that once were revolutionary and shunned, gained acceptance with time and became the norm. Innovations include the introduction of minimally invasive techniques, which decrease recovery times and surgical morbidity, while computer-assisted surgery has been shown to improve implant alignment and positioning. These innovations have not only improved precision in surgery but have also widened the application of knee replacement surgery to an ever-wider range of patients, including those suffering from complex deformity or comorbidity. Other improvements in the perioperative protocols, such as the adoption of a multimodal approach to pain management and accelerated rehabilitation programs, further facilitated the success and popularity of knee arthroplasty. These are complemented by the development of implant materials such as highly cross-linked polyethylene and improved ceramics, which have dramatically increased the longevity of prosthetic components and, by extension, reduced the rate of revision surgeries. Innovations in patient-specific instrumentation and preoperative planning, including 3D imaging and printing, have further refined the process, thus enabling highly customized procedures tailored to individual anatomical variations.

Total Knee Arthroplasty: The Progress

Till the introduction of robotics in arthroplasty, majors are taken to improve all aspects of TKA which affects its results, e.g., implant design, implant material, surgical technique, and radiological assessment. Nothing was changed with respect to except human-/surgeon-related factors. It is a paradigm shift toward integrating robotics into knee replacement surgery. As robotic-assisted surgery improved in terms of precision and accuracy, it reflects better alignment and positioning in prosthetic components. Navigation and imaging in advanced manners create a very detailed map of the patient's anatomical structure, thus allowing surgeons to perform procedures that are unparalleled in precision during planning and execution. Introduction of functional robotic arms eliminated the human-related errors as well. These devices are designed not to replace the surgeon but to assist in enhancing precision and efficiency.

ROBOTICS IN MEDICAL FIELD

The term "robot" originates from the Czech word "robota," meaning forced labor or activity. The concept was popularized in 1920 by Czech playwright Karel Čapek in his science fiction play *Rossum's Universal Robots*. In the play, robots are factory-manufactured artificial beings that perform routine tasks for humans. The play, which premiered on January 25, 1921, introduced the word "robot" to the English language and to the science fiction genre.

The first robot-assisted surgery took place in 1988, when robotic technology was used to perform neurosurgical biopsies. Since then, the use of robotics in surgery has expanded significantly.

Neurosurgery was the first specialty to adopt robotic technology, with the first recorded robotic surgery in 1988 for neurosurgical biopsies. Urosurgery followed in 1991 with robotic assistance in prostatic transurethral resection. Both specialties reported improved precision and fewer iatrogenic complications due to robotic assistance. Over time, robots have been incorporated into various surgical fields, offering benefits such as smaller incisions, increased precision in soft tissue management, faster recovery, quicker return to work, and reduced hospital stays.

Robotics in Orthopedics

The first robotic-assisted TKA was performed in 1988 in the United Kingdom, marking a significant milestone in the use of robotics in orthopedic surgery.

The integration of robotics into arthroplasty began in the late 20th century and has evolved rapidly. Below is a brief history of the development of robotic systems used in arthroplasty **(Table 2.1)**:

- *Early developments (1980s–1990s)*: The use of robotics in arthroplasty began with the goal of improving precision in joint replacement surgeries, particularly in procedures involving the hip and knee. Early robotic systems were conceptualized and developed in the 1980s and 1990s, often in conjunction with advancements in computer-aided surgery.

TABLE 2.1: History of the development of robotic systems used in arthroplasty.

Launch (year)	Robots	Company
1992	ROBODOC	Curexo Inc.
1990	CASPER	Ortho-Maquet/URS
2017	MAKO	Stryker
2017	NAVIO	Smith and Nephew
2020	ROSA	Zimmer–Biomet
2020	CUVIS	Curexo Inc.
2021	CORI	Smith and Nephew
2021	VELYS	DePuy Synthes
2024	MISSO	Meril Healthcare

CHAPTER 2: History of Robotics: The Evolution of Robotics in Modern Knee Replacements

- *1986*: Research and development for the surgical robot began in 1986 when IBM's Thomas J. Watson Research Center, and researchers at the University of California, Davis began a collaborative initiative of an innovative system for total hip arthroplasty (THA). Their goal was to create a robotic surgical system that would redefine precision joint replacement surgery. The *ROBODOC* prototype developed in 1989 was actually a modified version of an industrial robot. Its development was helped by Howard "Hap" Paul, a doctor of veterinary medicine, and Dr William Bargar, an orthopedic surgeon. In 1990, the system was first used to perform a total hip replacement on a dog with a congenital hip problem.
- *1992*: On November 7, 1992, a surgical team led by Dr Bargar at Sutter General Hospital, Sacramento, California, used ROBODOC to perform the *first robot-assisted human hip replacement*. So the first clinical use of a robotic system for joint replacement surgery occurred with the introduction of The ROBODOC System. Developed by Integrated Surgical Systems, ROBODOC was the first robotic-assisted system for performing THA. It was designed to assist surgeons in positioning the prosthetic components with high precision.
- *The CASPAR (Ortho-Maquet/URS, Schwerin, Germany)* was another early autonomous system. It was an image-guided, active robot used for THA and TKA similar to ROBODOC.
- *2017*: "*MAKO robotic system*" performed its robotic-assisted TKA in 2017. But the history starts in 1997. In 1997 Z-KAT company, founded by Rony Abovitz and other members, was developing a novel haptic robotic system for medical applications. Later it became MAKO Surgical Corp. and it developed the RAS (Robotic Arm Interactive System), which allowed for computer-assisted robotic surgery in both hip and knee arthroplasty. This system featured a robotic arm that helped surgeons in knee and hip replacements by improving precision in implant placement. The system was initially used for partial knee arthroplasty in 2006, followed by THA in 2008. In 2013, Stryker Orthopaedics took over MAKO surgical corp. Finally, MAKO robotic system performed its robotic-assisted TKA in 2017.
- *2017*: "*NAVIO Robotic systems*" was launched by smith and nephew in 2017. This was a hand held burr based system.
- *2020*: In 2020, "*ROSA knee robotic system*" was launched by Zimmer–Biomet. The original ROSA robot was designed for cranial operations and received U.S. Food and Drug Administration (FDA) clearance in 2012. Subsequently, the ROSA Spine edition was approved in 2016. In March 2019, the FDA approved an updated version of the robot, ROSA ONE Spine, for cranial and spinal applications. 2020 ROSA knee robot version of ROSA Spine, and has similar structural features as spine one robot.
- *2020*: The Korean company Curexo Inc. in 2020 launched a fully automated robotic system called "*CUVIS robotic system*". This was an image-based system with burr technology with active cutting by arm. Currently, the third generation of CUVIS robot is in the market. CUVIS robot is essentially an open system but in India it is closed for meril implants till now.
- *2021*: In 2021, Navio robotic system was replaced by "*CORI robotic system*" which is a more compact, surgeon-controlled, handheld robotic system. This

upgrade was offering faster passive infrared tracking camera and increased in cutting volumes compared to the previous system.
- *2021*: *VELYS™ Robotic-Assisted Solutions* (DePuy Synthes) got launched in 2021. This is a saw-based imageless system. Later based on same platform in 2024, VELYS spine robot is launched.
- *2024*: In 2024, the *"MISSO Robotic System"* developed by Meril Healthcare Pvt Ltd is launched. It is the first robot indigenously developed in India and is a fully active surgical robot with image based system. It works with burr technology with active cutting by arm.

It is a paradigm shift toward integrating robotics into knee replacement surgery. As robotic-assisted surgery improved in terms of precision and accuracy, it reflects better alignment and positioning in prosthetic components. This robotic world is advancing and upgrading very rapidly.

CONCLUSION

The journey of TKA from an underperforming surgical procedure to one of the most successful and transformative operations in modern medicine is a testament to relentless innovation and scientific pursuit. What began in the shadows of hip replacement surgery has now emerged into a highly sophisticated and precision-driven field—thanks to the exponential growth of robotic technology in orthopedics.

From the early days when inconsistent implant designs, poor understanding of knee biomechanics, and limited surgical standardization plagued outcomes, we have come a long way. The steady evolution of surgical instruments, implant materials, perioperative protocols, and alignment philosophies laid a strong foundation. But it was the integration of robotics that truly redefined precision, repeatability, and personalization in knee arthroplasty.

The history of robotics in TKA is both fascinating and inspiring. It mirrors the evolution of modern surgery itself—starting from primitive, bulky robotic systems such as ROBODOC and CASPAR, which were groundbreaking in their time, to the sleek, surgeon-friendly, data-driven robotic platforms such as MAKO, ROSA, CORI, and India's own MISSO robot. Each generation brought a leap in accuracy, adaptability, and clinical outcomes.

These robots were never meant to replace the surgeon but to empower them—to eliminate human errors, to overcome anatomical variations, to address challenging deformities with confidence, and to ensure that the optimal plan becomes a reality with submillimeter accuracy. The transformation is not merely technological but philosophical, shifting from "one-size-fits-all" to "patient-specific precision."

Robotics today plays a pivotal role in every phase of TKA—from preoperative planning and intraoperative execution to postoperative analytics. Image-based planning, haptic feedback, active cutting arms, and real-time ligament balancing have taken the guesswork out of surgery. For patients, this translates to smaller incisions, faster recovery, lower complication rates, and superior long-term satisfaction.

CHAPTER 2: History of Robotics: The Evolution of Robotics in Modern Knee Replacements

As robotic systems continue to evolve and newer platforms emerge—like the fully indigenized MISSO system—accessibility and affordability are also improving. The future of robotic arthroplasty lies not only in refining surgical precision but also in democratizing it, ensuring that cutting-edge care is available to all strata of society.

In conclusion, the evolution of robotics in TKA is not merely a technological achievement; it is a paradigm shift in how we think, plan, and perform joint replacement surgeries. It reflects the surgical community's commitment to continuous improvement and sets the stage for the next era of smart, connected, and outcome-driven orthopedic care.

The journey is far from over. As robotics intertwines with artificial intelligence, machine learning, and predictive analytics, the next chapters in this exciting story promise to be even more transformative—for the surgeon, for the patient, and for the science of orthopedics itself.

CHAPTER 3

Alignment Strategies in Total Knee Arthroplasty

Pramod Bhor, Sourabh Kulkarni, Sunil Shetty, Sawankumar Pawar, Syed Mussadique Ali

▊ INTRODUCTION

Total knee arthroplasty (TKA) is a frequently performed orthopedic procedure aimed at alleviating pain and improving function in patients with severe osteoarthritis. A pivotal aspect of successful TKA is the alignment of the femoral and tibial components, which significantly influences functional outcomes and implant longevity. Over the period, different alignment philosophies have emerged, challenging the traditional gold standard of mechanical alignment (MA). This chapter will explore the various alignment strategies currently employed in TKA, outlining their principles, potential benefits, and limitations based on the available literature.

▊ MECHANICAL ALIGNMENT

Mechanical alignment is a traditional and widely used technique in TKA. The primary objective of MA is to reconstruct the limb with a neutral mechanical axis, aiming for a hip-knee-ankle (HKA) angle of 180°.

Principle

The rationale behind MA is to create a horizontal joint line and a neutral mechanical axis, which is believed to provide evenly distributed load across the implant-bone interface and provide the best mechanical environment for prosthetic longevity by minimizing laterally directed ground reaction forces. Surgeons often employ either measured resection or gap balancing techniques to achieve balanced medial-lateral soft-tissue tension and equal flexion-extension gaps.

Component Positioning

Hip-knee-ankle angle of 180° is achieved by positioning both the femoral and tibial components perpendicular to the mechanical axes of their respective bones in the coronal plane **(Figs. 3.1A and B)**.

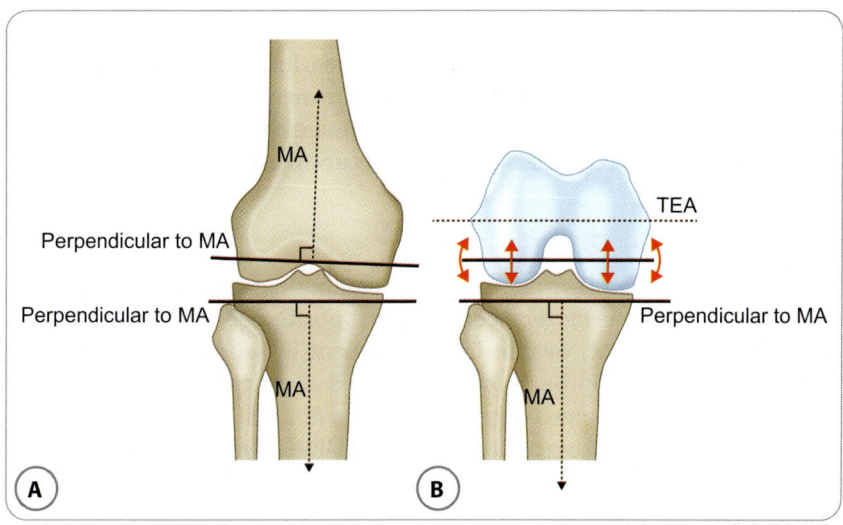

FIGS. 3.1A AND B: Mechanical alignment (MA).
(TEA: transepicondylar axis)

Joint Line Inclination

The natural knee has a slightly oblique joint line, typically 2–3° of varus in relation to the mechanical axis. But when both the components are put perpendicular to their respective mechanical axis the resulting joint line orientation angle (JLOA) is usually shifts to valgus than natural knee.

Challenges

Despite of its long-term survivorship, MA has been criticized for disregarding patient-specific knee joint anatomy and constitutional alignment, as implants are consistently placed in the same manner for every patient. This can lead to potential problems such as lateral column lengthening, distal femoral prosthetic overstuffing, increased patellofemoral retinacular tension, and altered native knee kinematics. Furthermore, some patients remain dissatisfied after mechanically aligned with functional outcomes proving inconsistent. Studies have shown that the native limb alignment in nonosteoarthritic individuals often deviates from a perfectly neutral 180°.

ANATOMIC ALIGNMENT

Anatomic alignment (AA) for TKAs was originally described by Hungerford and Krackow. The AA technique strives to achieve a neutral HKA angle while respecting the anatomical joint line orientation of 2–3° from the horizontal, aiming to bring the joint line parallel to the floor during a single leg stance. It attempts to replicate the anatomical alignment of the knee before the onset of osteoarthritis.

Principle

Anatomical alignment seeks to recreate the prearthritic knee's configuration, including the normal joint line inclination and the mechanical axis. The goal is to replicate the natural knee's mechanics and soft tissue balance, potentially leading to improved functional outcomes and implant survivorship.

Component Positioning

In achieving anatomical alignment, the tibial component is positioned with a 2–3° varus angulation, and the femoral component is positioned with a corresponding valgus angulation. Hence, overall limb alignment is neutral with joint line in natural obliquity. This approach often involves a slight varus positioning of the tibial component and a valgus positioning of the femoral component relative to the mechanical axis, resulting in an oblique joint line **(Figs. 3.2A and B)**.

Joint Line Inclination

The natural knee has a slightly oblique joint line, typically 2–3° of varus in relation to the mechanical axis. Anatomical alignment aims to reproduce this obliquity.

Benefits

By replicating the natural knee's alignment, anatomical alignment may lead to better soft tissue balance, improved knee mechanics, and potentially better functional outcomes after TKA. In knee arthroplasty, anatomical alignment aims to restore the knee's predisease alignment and geometry, including the natural joint line and mechanical axis.

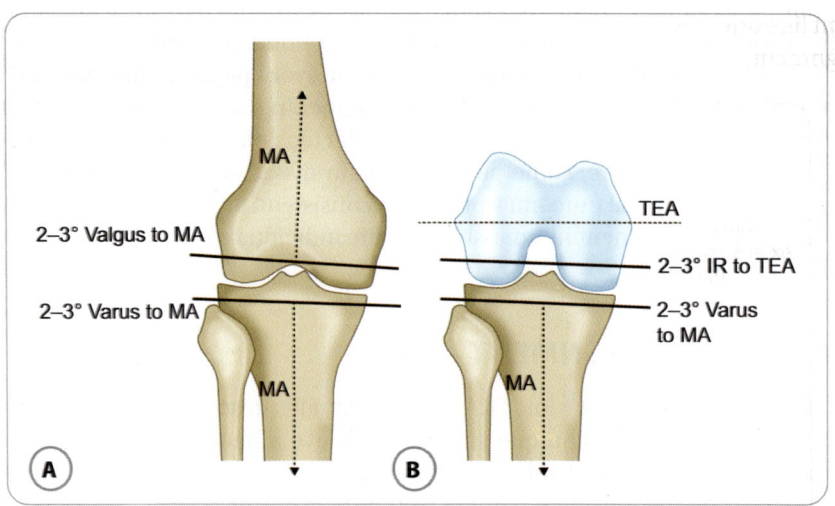

FIGS. 3.2A AND B: Anatomical alignment.
(MA: mechanical alignment; TEA: transepicondylar axis)

Challenges

While promising, achieving accurate anatomical alignment can be challenging due to individual variations in knee anatomy and the difficulty in replicating the exact predisease configuration.

■ KINEMATIC ALIGNMENT

Kinematic alignment was described by Howell et al. KA is an "individualized" or patient-specific technique that aims for knee resurfacing with restitution of the prearthritic anatomy and preservation of the soft-tissue envelope.

Principle

The principle of KA is to resurface the femur maintaining the native femoral joint line obliquity (JLO) and balance the flexion and extension gaps with tibial resection. KA respects the three kinematic axes of the knee with respect to the joint lines of the posterior and distal femur and proximal tibia.

Component Positioning

As the principle of KA is to resurface the femur maintaining the native femoral JLO, the femoral component is put precisely at the native distal femoral joint line. So the medial and lateral distal femoral cuts are the same and are matching the thickness of the implant. KA aims to achieve symmetrical posterior condylar resections of the distal femur after correcting for cartilage wear, placing the implant in a native, rotationally neutral position. Then the balancing of the flexion and extension gaps is achieved with tibial resection **(Figs. 3.3A and B)**.

Joint Line Inclination

Joint line orientation angle in KA may remain between native valgus to the neutral alignment.

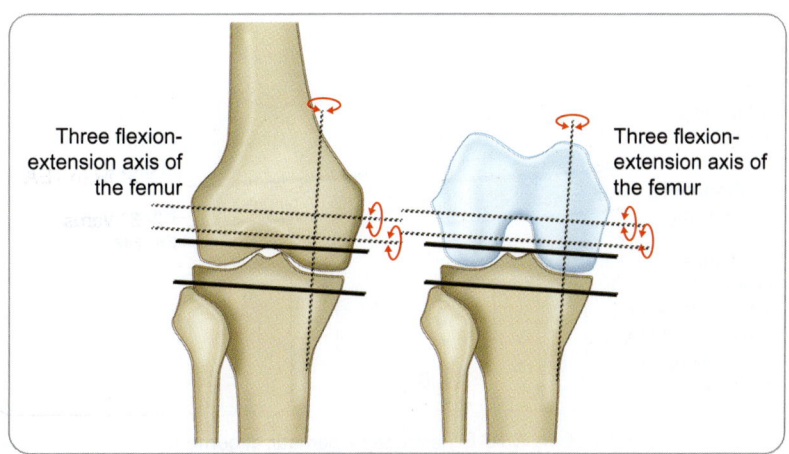

FIGS. 3.3A AND B: Kinematic alignment.

Benefits

Proponents of KA believe this strategy may require less soft tissue release, preserve bone, reduce postoperative pain, and improve postoperative function, thereby reducing patient discontent. Some studies suggest KA may better reproduce normal gait and natural tibiofemoral kinematics compared to MA. It may also reduce the knee adduction moment. Compared to MA, KA for osteoarthritic patients with slight to mid constitutional knee frontal deformity may enable a faster recovery and generally generate higher functional TKA outcomes at early to mid-term.

Challenges

Some authors have noted potential concerns regarding implant survival and function in the long term with KA, particularly in varus knees longer follow-up is needed to assess its long-term outcomes.

RESTRICTED KINEMATIC ALIGNMENT

Restricted KA (rKA) is a TKA technique that aims to restore native knee kinematics while avoiding extreme anatomical modifications as suggested in KA. Hence rKA represents a compromise between MA and true KA.

Principle (Safe Zone)

It limits the femoral and tibial prosthesis coronal alignment within a safe range, typically ±5° of neutral, and the overall combined lower limb coronal orientation within ±3° of neutral. This approach offers a compromise between "true" KA and MA, according to a study published on the NCBI.

Adjustment of coronal limb alignment and JLO is primarily achieved by fine-tuning the tibial component positioning **(Figs. 3.4A and B)**.

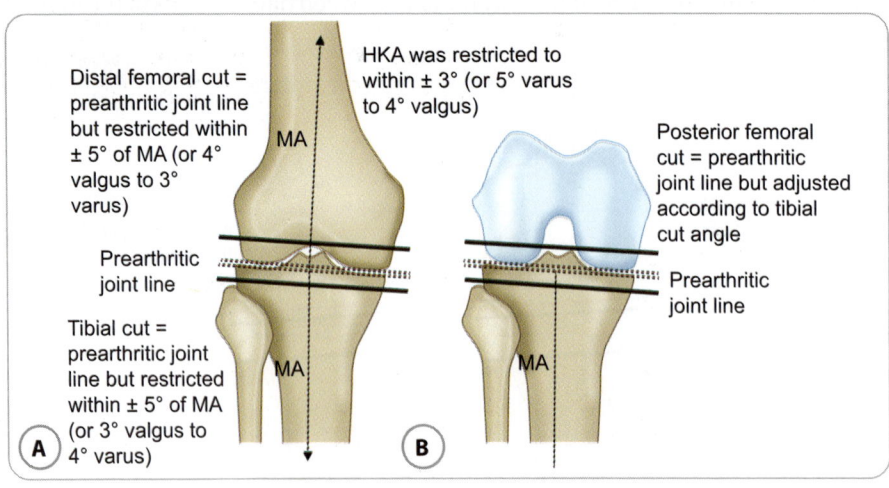

FIGS. 3.4A AND B: Restricted kinematic alignment.
(HKA: hip-knee-ankle; MA: mechanical alignment)

Benefits

Unlike adjusted MA (aMA), rKA follows the main technical principle of KA, respecting the KA of the femoral component as much as possible. Restricted KA generally leads to better gap balance and lower pressure differences compared to MA, as well as improved knee balance. On the other side as rKA limits the degree to which the prosthesis can be aligned in varus or valgus, which can help prevent implant failure and other complications. rKA often requires minimal anatomical modifications and ligamentous releases compared to MA, making it a less invasive procedure.

Challenges

The rKA needs computerized navigation or robotic navigation to achieve rKA.

ADJUSTED MECHANICAL ALIGNMENT

Adjusted MA represents another alternative to traditional MA. While still aiming for a mechanically aligned limb, aMA allows for minor adjustments to component positioning based on intraoperative findings, particularly concerning soft tissue balance. Conversely with rKA, bone cut adjustment in aMA is performed to bring the patient in their safe zone of alignment, potentially requiring substantial bone cut (tibial or/and femoral) adjustment.

Functional/Mixed/Hybrid Alignment

Functional alignment (FA) is described as an evolution of KA enabled by advancements in technology, particularly robotic-assisted systems. This approach involves manipulating alignment, bone resections, soft tissue releases, and/or implant positioning using robotic assistance to optimize TKA function for a patient's specific alignment, bone morphology, and soft tissue envelope. FA aims to restore native knee kinematics and improve functional outcomes. It often involves 3D planning of the femoral and tibial prostheses prior to bone resection, with soft tissue balance assessed using sensors or surgeon feel, and adjustments made using 3D planning software.

Implant Positioning

The femoral component is typically adjusted from a starting point aligned with the mechanical axis to balance the extension gap, and its rotation is set within ±3° of the surgical transepicondylar axis to balance the flexion gap. The tibial component is aligned to the tibial mechanical axis and then modified within 0–3° varus to balance the flexion and extension gaps, matching the patient's native posterior tibial slope. So in FA femur remains perpendicular to the femoral mechanical axis but the tibial component is adjusted to within ±3° for better ligament balancing (**Figs. 3.5A and B**).

Benefits

Studies suggest that FA with robotic assistance may lead to better patient-reported outcomes compared to manual MA due to better ligament balancing, minimal soft tissue release and more natural JLOA.

■ INVERSE KINEMATIC ALIGNMENT

The principle of inverse KA is to resurface the tibia and to make gap balancing by adjusting femoral implant placement. This results in similar medial and lateral bone resections of proximal tibia to maintain the native tibial JLO and gap balancing is then performed by adjusting the femoral resections **(Figs. 3.6A and B)**.

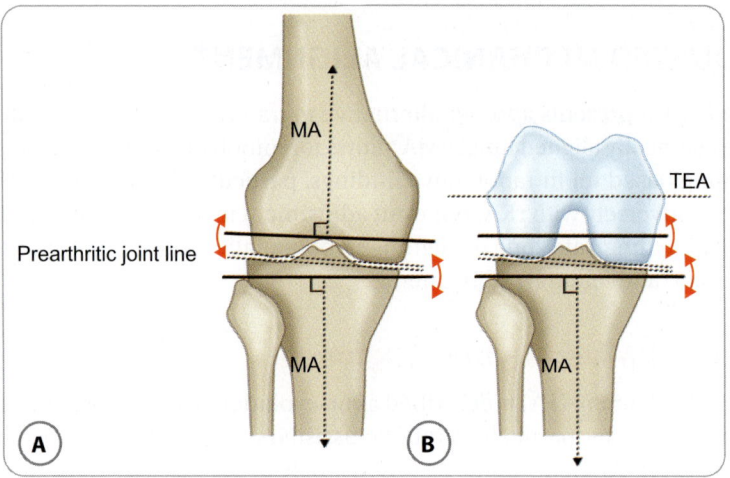

FIGS. 3.5A AND B: Functional alignment.

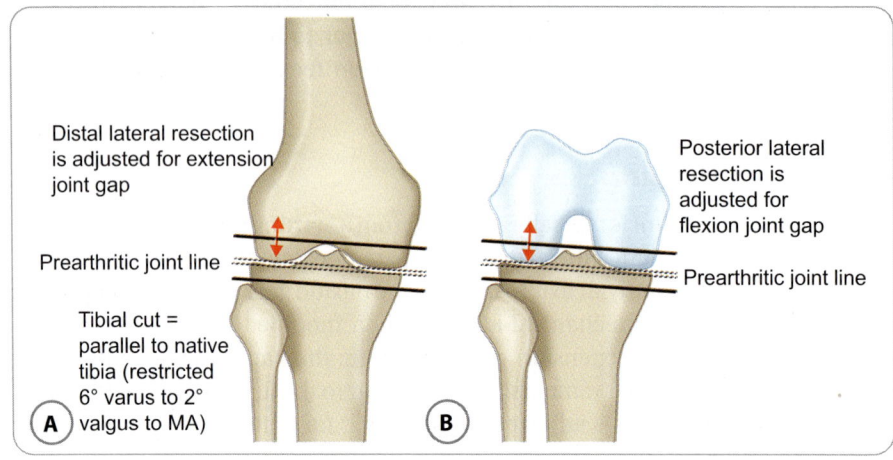

FIGS. 3.6A AND B: Inverse kinematic alignment.

# THE CORONAL PLANE ALIGNMENT OF THE KNEE CLASSIFICATION AND ITS IMPACT ON ALIGNMENT STRATEGIES IN TOTAL KNEE ARTHROPLASTY

The coronal plane alignment of the knee (CPAK) classification has emerged as a valuable tool for understanding knee phenotypes and guiding the selection of appropriate alignment strategies.

The CPAK classification was proposed by MacDessi et al. in 2021. It offers a pragmatic and comprehensive system for describing coronal knee alignment in both healthy and arthritic knees. Unlike simpler classifications that focus solely on the HKA angle, CPAK incorporates two independent variables:

Arithmetic Hip-knee-ankle Angle

This estimates the constitutional limb alignment (varus, neutral, or valgus) and is calculated as the medial proximal tibial angle (MPTA) minus the lateral distal femoral angle (LDFA). A negative aHKA indicates varus, a positive value indicates valgus, and a value around zero indicates neutral constitutional alignment. Importantly, aHKA is not affected by joint space narrowing or tibiofemoral subluxation **(Figs. 3.7A to C)**.

Joint Line Obliquity

This describes the orientation of the joint line relative to the floor in double leg stance. It is calculated as the sum of MPTA and LDFA. CPAK categorizes JLO as **(Figs. 3.8A to B)**:
- Apex distal (MPTA + LDFA < 177°),
- Neutral (MPTA + LDFA 177° to 183° inclusive), or
- Apex proximal (MPTA + LDFA > 183°).

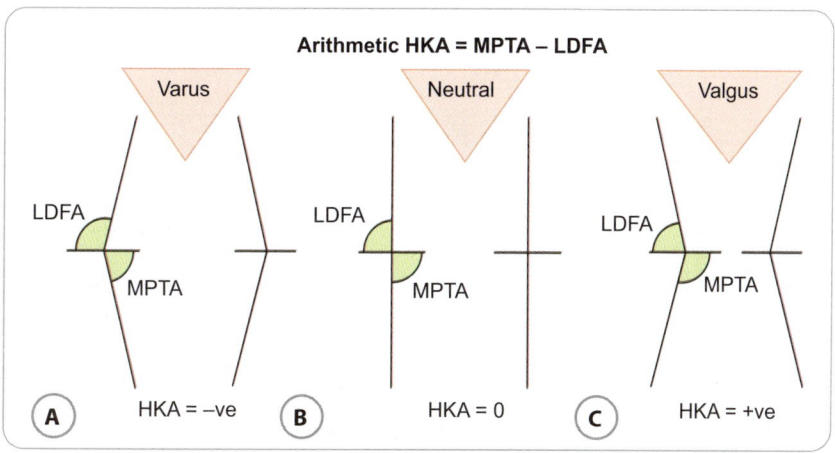

FIGS. 3.7A TO C: Arithmetic hip-knee-ankle angle.

PHENOTYPE CLASSIFICATION

This terminology avoids the ambiguity of using "varus" and "valgus" for both limb alignment and joint line orientation.

By combining the three subgroups of aHKA (varus, neutral, and valgus) with the three subgroups of JLO (apex distal, neutral, and apex proximal) in a matrix, the CPAK classification defines nine distinct knee phenotypes. These phenotypes provide a better understanding of coronal knee alignment beyond simple varus, neutral, or valgus limb alignment **(Fig. 3.9)**.

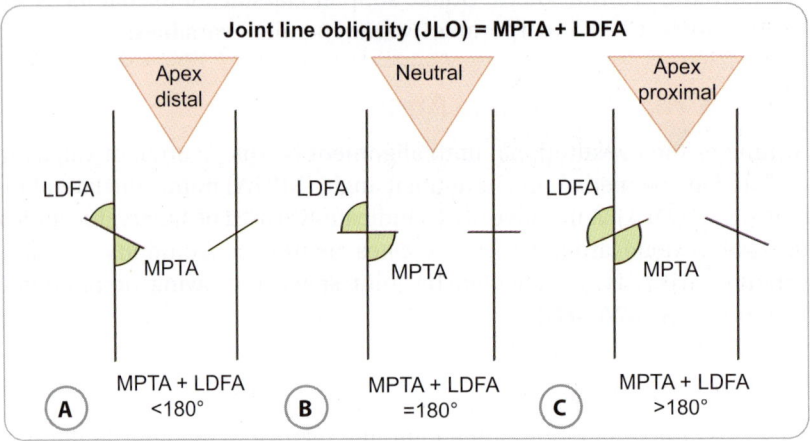

FIGS. 3.8A TO C: Joint line obliquity.
(MPTA: medial proximal tibial angle; LDFA: lateral distal femoral angle)

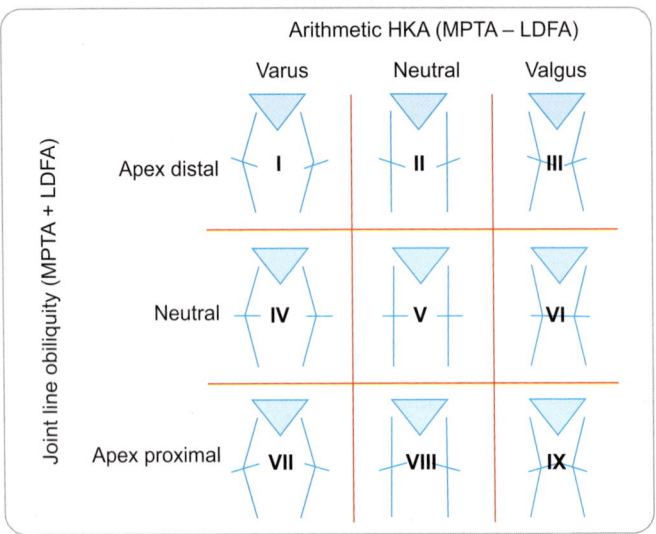

FIG 3.9: CPAK Classification.
(CPAK: coronal plane alignment of the knee; MPTA: medial proximal tibial angle; LDFA: lateral distal femoral angle)

APPLICABILITY OF CPAK IN HEALTHY AND OSTEOARTHRITIC KNEES

A key strength of the CPAK classification is its applicability to both healthy and osteoarthritic populations. Studies have shown similar frequency distributions across all nine CPAK types when comparing healthy volunteers and patients with osteoarthritis. The most common categories observed were type II (neutral aHKA, apex distal JLO), type I (varus aHKA, apex distal JLO), and type V (neutral aHKA, neutral JLO). Notably, CPAK type V, representing the target for traditional MA (neutral limb alignment with neutral JLO), only accounted for a small proportion of both populations. This observation challenges the notion that a neutral mechanical axis with a neutral joint line is representative of the majority of knees.

CPAK AND ITS INFLUENCE ON ALIGNMENT STRATEGIES

The CPAK classification provides a framework for considering more patient-specific alignment strategies in TKA. By categorizing knees based on their constitutional alignment and JLO, surgeons can move beyond a purely systematic approach such as MA and consider techniques that aim to restore or respect the patient's native anatomy. CPAK can help determine whether a patient might be a candidate for:

- *Mechanical alignment*: Traditionally aimed at achieving CPAK type V (neutral aHKA, neutral JLO). However, given the low prevalence of this phenotype, MA may lead to a nonphysiological alignment in many other patients.
- *Anatomic alignment*: The study suggests that CPAK type II (neutral aHKA and apex distal JLO) aligns with the principles described for AA.
- *Kinematic alignment*: CPAK can help identify knee phenotypes that may benefit most from KA when the optimization of soft tissue balance is prioritized. A study comparing intraoperative soft tissue balance in computer-assisted TKAs randomized to KA or MA within each CPAK type revealed that a greater proportion of KA TKAs achieved optimal balance across all CPAK types compared to MA.

Overall, The CPAK classification represents a valuable step toward a more personalized approach to alignment in TKA. By providing a simple and comprehensive system for describing coronal knee alignment based on constitutional limb alignment (aHKA) and JLO, CPAK allows surgeons to better understand the underlying knee phenotype. Evidence suggests that CPAK can help predict which patients are more likely to benefit from KA in terms of achieving optimal soft tissue balance and potentially reducing the need for aggressive bone recuts compared to traditional MA.

CONCLUSION

The field of TKA is continuously evolving, with a growing recognition that a "one-size-fits-all" approach to alignment may not be optimal for all patients. While

MA has a strong history of implant survival, alternative, more personalized alignment strategies such as kinematic, restricted kinematic, and FA are gaining traction due to their potential to improve functional outcomes and restore more natural knee kinematics. The choice of alignment strategy is influenced by various factors, including the patient's prearthritic anatomy, the degree of deformity, and the surgeon's experience and preference. Advanced technologies such as robotic-assisted surgery are playing an increasingly important role in facilitating these personalized alignment strategies and optimizing surgical outcomes.

Components of Robotic System

*Sourabh Kulkarni, Pramod Bhor,
Sachin Yashwant Kale, Arvind Vatkar*

INTRODUCTION

Each of these arthroplasty robotic systems are complex machines. They are a beautiful example of integration between advanced software and hardware. These robotic systems are made up of four parts:
1. Optical tracking system (OTS)
2. Robotic arm
3. Cutting tool
4. Interactive device (screen or monitor)

OPTICAL TRACKING SYSTEM

Navigation is an integral part of all robotic systems. Navigation helps in tracking surgical tools, bones, and implants. OTS is an important component of surgical navigation systems, where it can provide measurement data for real-time surgical tool tracking. These optical trackers deliver reliable measurement data with submillimeter accuracy.

When integrated into the workflow of surgical navigation systems, the optical tracker acts as the link between patient image sets and the physical 3D space. It enables the positions and orientations of surgical tools to be instantly localized and visualized within the operative field. Multiple tools can be tracked at once without interrupting the surgical workflow.

Key Components

Optical Cameras

NDI cameras work on the principle of infrared light. They have both infrared light transmitter and receiver. The infrared light reflected from a specifically designed reflective marker is captured in the camera **(Fig. 4.1)**.

High-speed cameras track the trackers having highly reflective markers. These cameras are mounted in the operating room, typically positioned above the surgical field. Depending upon their capture angles, minimum distance between camera and surgical field is decided.

Reflective Markers (Tracker Balls)

In general, two types of markers are used in the OTS—(1) passive and (2) active. Active markers generate infrared light by their own. Hence, they need a power source. On the other hand, passive markers need an infrared light source from the camera. Reflected light from these markers is used for tracking. So, they do not need a power source. Hence in all surgical robots, passive markers are used.

These passive markers are of three types:
1. *Sphere*: Spherical shape of these markers makes them easier to identify at various angles. These markers are used in CUVIS and MISSO robotic systems **(Fig. 4.2)**.
2. *Glass lenses*: Glass lens marker is a passive, retroreflective, and wipeable lens. These markers are used in VELYS robotic system **(Fig. 4.3)**.
3. *Flat markers*: These are flat-shaped reflective markers used in Rosa, Cori, and Mako robotic systems.

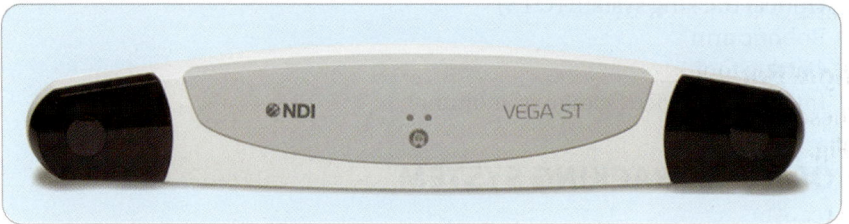

FIG. 4.1: NDI optical camera.

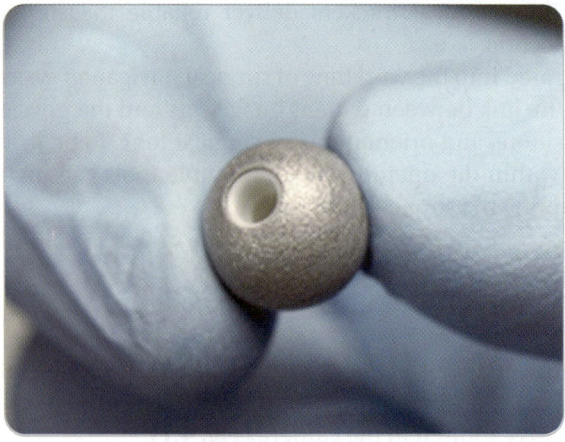

FIG. 4.2: Spherical marker.

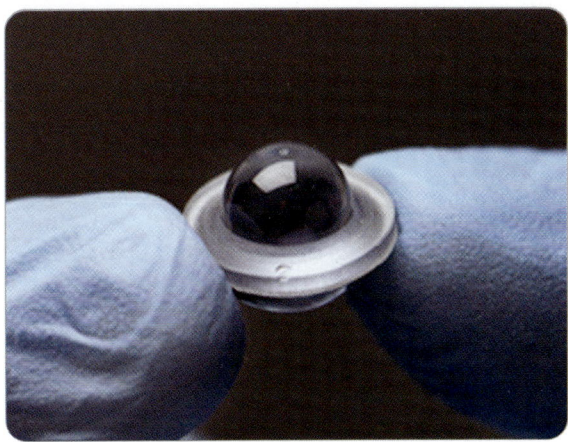

FIG. 4.3: Glass marker.

Such markers have a high reflectivity index. The markers are combined in a plane in a unique configuration that helps to define a plane. Markers arranged in a plane are then further used to track rigid body motion of the objects under consideration in real-time. Hence, the entire system including the camera and markers is called the OTS.

Rigid Body Tools (Tracker Frames)

These are rigid frames on which multiple reflective markers are attached **(Fig. 4.4)**.

Geometric configuration of these markers collectively form a unit which helps in real-time tracking of the object on which it is mounted.

Such five to six markers are assigned to the femur, tibia probe, calibration tool, and robot **(Figs. 4.5A and B)**. These in turn track movements of each component in the operation theater intraoperatively.

Data of femoral anatomy and spatial orientation is added to the software with respect to the femoral marker tool. Hence, varus valgus and angular movements of femur can be measured by equivalent respective movement of femoral marker tool.

This information is displayed to the surgeon in the form of a 3D model of the patient's knee on a screen, guiding them through each step.

Pins

These are the Steinman pins used for mounting the femoral and tibial marker. These are rigid, autoclavable, and partially threaded stainless steel (SS) pins. Various robotic systems use pins with different diameters: Thinnest being 3.2 mm to thickest being 4 mm.

There are also 5-mm diameter SS pins which are used in fully automated systems to fix femur and tibia to the robot to stabilize them in the cutting process.

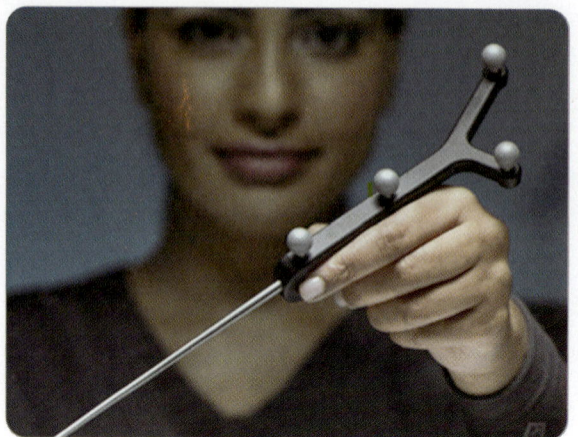

FIG. 4.4: Probe tracker frame.

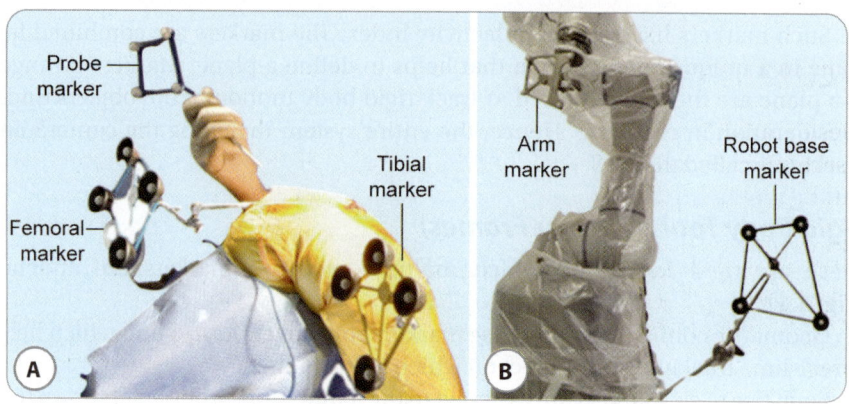

FIGS. 4.5A AND B: Various markers in robotic surgery.

ROBOTIC ARM

The robotic arm is the main output device which controls the precision in robotic surgery. Usually, these robotic arms have six-axis design for precise maneuverability **(Fig. 4.6)**. Six-axis design means it has six joints through which the robot can articulate to achieve fine movements. This six-axis design provides flexibility to reach complex angles during surgery and enables accurate positioning of cutting tools. This robotic arm has precise positional accuracy. Working radius, arm lengths, and range of motion at each joint vary between different companies. As per individual systems, these arms control the cutting tool except few.

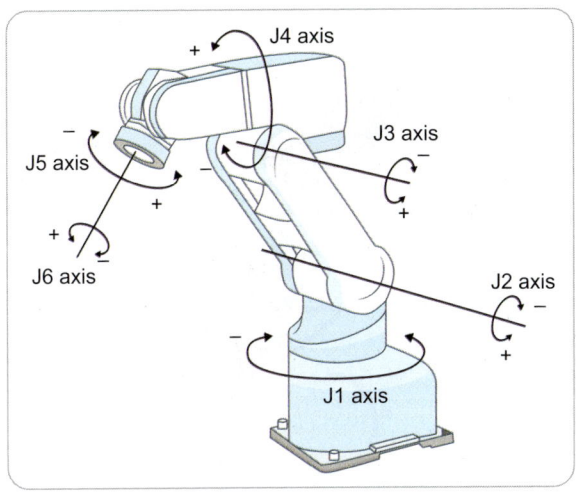

FIG. 4.6: Robotic arm with six axes.

CUTTING TOOLS

These are the tools which help the surgeon or the robotic arm to perform bone resection with precision within desired range. Few robotic systems don't have cutting tools in their system, e.g., ROSA.

These cutting tools can be either saw based or burr based.
- *Saw system*: Oscillating or rotary saws are designed for controlled bone cutting. MAKO and VELYS systems use this type of tool **(Fig. 4.7)**.
- *Burr systems*: High-speed burrs are used for milling the bone at desired level. CUVIS, MISSO, and CORI systems use this type of tool **(Fig. 4.8)**.
Some of these cutting tools are equipped with *haptic feedback* sensors. Haptic feedback is the reciprocal resistance force generated by the bone sensed by a cutting tool. This sensory information is used to ensure the cutting tool is in the bony boundaries. This is a great safety feature. It also detects pressure applied by the arm and halts cutting if resistance is too high or if the arm deviates from the surgical plan.

Cooling System

In automated burring systems due to high-speed milling, a greater amount of heat is generated which is harmful for bone tissue. Hence in these systems water irrigation systems are provided to prevent overheating and bone necrosis during the cutting process.

INTERACTIVE DEVICE (SCREEN OR MONITOR)

These are audio visual output devices which help the surgeon understand the real time information provided by the navigation system **(Fig. 4.9)**.

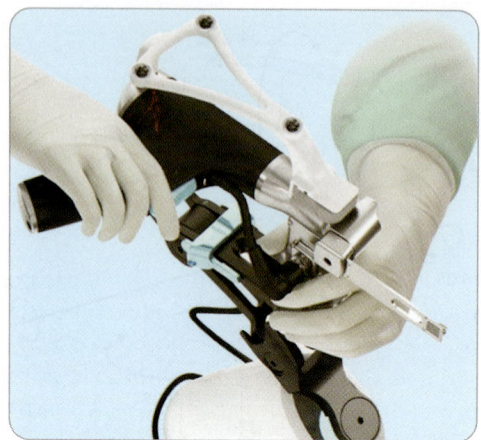

FIG. 4.7: Saw-based system.

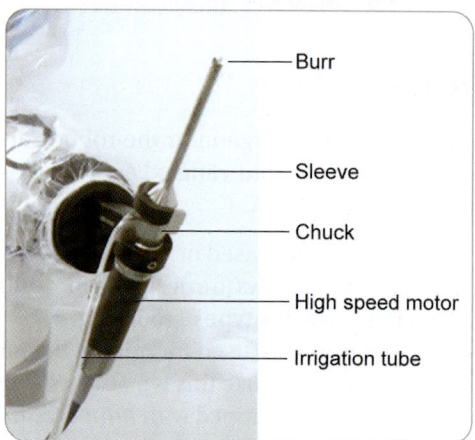

FIG. 4.8: Burr-based system.

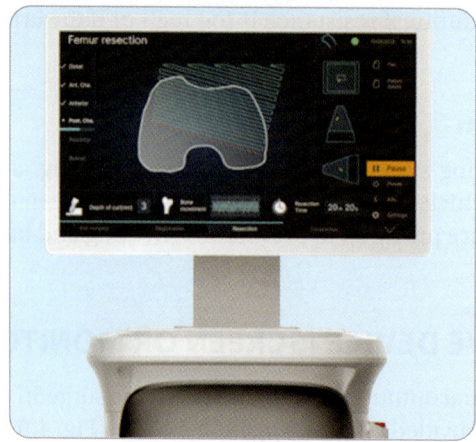

FIG. 4.9: Interactive screen.

Usually, these are medical grade monitors. Few of them are touch screen monitors.

All these robots have at least two central processing units. These CPUs are packed under the robot cart and screen cart.

CONCLUSION

Modern robotic systems used in arthroplasty are a seamless blend of advanced engineering and medical precision. They bring together highly specialized components that work in perfect synergy to enhance surgical accuracy, safety, and outcomes. The OTS forms the backbone of surgical navigation, enabling real-time spatial tracking of tools and anatomy with submillimeter accuracy. The robotic arm, with its multiaxis articulation, brings precision, and repeatability to complex surgical maneuvers. The cutting tools, whether saw-based or burr-driven, are designed for controlled and safe bone resections, often aided by haptic feedback and cooling systems to preserve tissue health. Finally, the interactive interface—the surgeon's window into the robotic system—displays critical information and guides decision-making in real time.

Each component plays a vital role, but it is their integration that transforms robotic arthroplasty into a cutting-edge solution in orthopedic surgery. Understanding these components provides the foundation for appreciating the technology's capabilities and helps surgeons utilize robotic systems more effectively and confidently.

Classification of Robotic Systems

Sourabh Kulkarni, Pramod Bhor,
Sachin Yashwant Kale, Vishal Kumar

INTRODUCTION

Robotic systems can be divided in multiple categories based on functionality and working processes.
- *Requirement of preoperative imaging*:
  - Image based
  - Imageless
- *Functionality of robotic arm in cutting process*:
  - Passive robotic arm
  - Semiactive robotic arm
  - Active robotic arm
- *Implant choice availability*:
  - Open platform system
  - Closed platform system

IMAGE-BASED VERSUS IMAGELESS SYSTEMS

Image-based Systems

In these systems, preoperative imaging is utilized for planning surgery and implant placement. There are two types of image-based processing systems:
1. *CT scan based*: CT scan images are processed within the software preoperatively to get a three-dimensional (3D) model of leg from hip–knee to ankle. This information is utilized to identify bone resection depth, preoperative and target postoperative alignment, optimal component size and alignment, leg length and offset restoration, volumetric bone removal, deformity correction, and the haptic boundaries of hard tissue removal, e.g., *CUVIS, MISSO, and MAKO* robotic systems.
2. *X-ray based*: Some systems utilize anteroposterior and lateral X-ray views of knee to form a virtual 3D model of affected knee which helps in planning implant intraoperatively. It helps in knowing implant size preoperatively but

implant alignment planning is not possible (preoperatively) in this system as hip center and ankle center are not available, e.g., *ROSA* robotic system.

Imageless Systems

Imageless systems rely on registration of the patient anatomy after surgical exposure in the operating room to create a virtual model and surgical plan that is then executed during the procedure.
- *Pros*: No need of CT and logistically easier.
- *Cons*: Precision in acquiring anatomy is less than image-based systems.

BASED ON ROBOTIC ARM CUTTING PROCESS

Passive System

In this system, the cutting tool is not in the robot's arm nor does it control the cutting tool. Here, the robot will hold a cutting zig at a determined level and the surgeon has to cut bone traditionally with a handheld saw system, i.e., *ROSA*.
- *Advantages*: Surgeons preference to hold saw and cut the bone is retained.
- *Disadvantages*: Human hand cutting error, instrument-based error is not rectified.

Semiactive

In this system, cutting tools are in the robot's arm but will not be advanced by the robot. Surgeon has to hold the cutting tool and has to advance it on the bone, i.e., *Mako* and VELYS.

Another version in this class is cutting tool is not in the robot's hand but is controlled by robotic software, i.e., *CORI*.
- *Advantages*: Surgeons preference to hold saw and cut the bone is retained.
- *Disadvantages*: Human hand versus robotic arm struggle is noticed.

Active

In this system, cutting tool is in robot's arm and also robotic arm will control and advance this cutting tool without surgeon's interference, i.e., *CUVIS* and *MISSO*.
- *Advantages*: Human hand cutting error, instrument-based error is taken care of.
- *Disadvantages*: Precision in surgical methodology is required.

TROCCAZ CLASSIFICATION

In literature, we found one classification suggested by J. Troccaz in 2001 **(Fig. 5.1)**.

CLOSED VERSUS OPEN PLATFORMS

- *Closed systems*: Implant platforms allowing only one specific manufacturer's implant(s) to be utilized during the procedure. Currently in India, all robotic systems are closed systems.

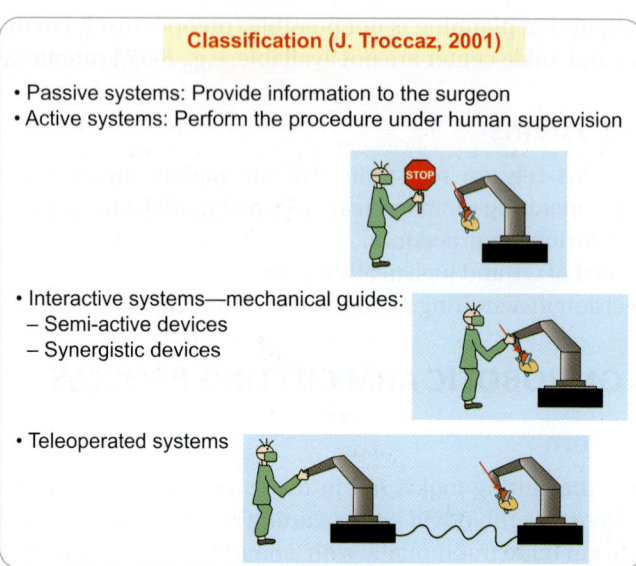

FIG. 5.1: Troccaz classification.

- *Open systems*: Implant platforms can allow different implant companies and designs to be utilized per the surgeon's preference or patient's demand.

CONCLUSION

Robotic systems in arthroplasty can be classified in various ways, each influencing surgical planning, execution, and outcomes. The distinction between image-based and imageless systems highlights the trade-off between preoperative precision and intraoperative convenience. While image-based systems offer superior accuracy through detailed 3D planning, imageless systems simplify logistics without compromising functionality for many standard cases.

Classification based on the functionality of the robotic arm—from passive to active—shows the evolution of control and precision. Passive systems rely entirely on the surgeon's skill, while active systems represent the peak of automation, minimizing human error. Semiactive systems strike a balance, integrating surgeon control with robotic accuracy.

The third category, implant platform type, determines flexibility. While closed platforms currently dominate the Indian market, offering tight integration and reliability, open platforms promise greater freedom, and adaptability in implant choices in the future.

Understanding these classifications is essential for orthopedic surgeons to select the right robotic system tailored to their surgical style, patient needs, and institutional infrastructure. This classification lays the foundation for evaluating the strengths and limitations of each robotic system in clinical practice.

CUVIS Joint Robotic System

*Pramod Bhor, Sawankumar Pawar, Sachin Yashwant Kale,
Sourabh Kulkarni, Syed Mussadique Ali, Raj M Sawant*

INTRODUCTION

CUVIS joint is a fully automated image-based robotic system. It is equipped with a 6-axis arm with a milling device and an optical tracking system (OTS). CUVIS joint robotic system is an advanced system capable of three-dimensional (3D) preplanning and precise cutting to provide accurate component sizes preoperatively and help surgeons minimize errors and to improve implant components' position and patient outcomes results. India's leading orthopedic implant manufacturer, Meril Healthcare Private Limited, in collaboration with South Korea-based Curexo Inc., brought this technology to India to enhance the quality of innovative orthopedic and rehabilitation robotics systems. The CUVIS Joint robotic system is designed on the basis of four core values: Accuracy, flexibility, safety, and ease of use. With the help of patients' specific computed tomography (CT) imaging, the surgeon and team will do the preplanning of surgery a day prior with the planning device. The main console with an OTS helps with the real-time monitoring and guides the surgeon with the execution. A robotic arm with a milling tool mounted on its tip does the most important work of bone cutting.

COMPONENT OF CUVIS SYSTEM

CUVIS joint primarily has three major components **(Fig. 6.1)**: Main console, robotic arm, and planning device. With the help of patients' specific CT imaging, the surgeon and team will do the preplanning of surgery a day prior with the planning device. The main console with an OTS helps with the real-time monitoring and guides the surgeon with the execution.

A robotic arm with a milling tool mounted on its tip does the most important work of bone cutting.

Main Console

Equipped with an OTS camera holder and a monitor to guide the surgical procedure. It is the main component used to guide the entire system in conjunction

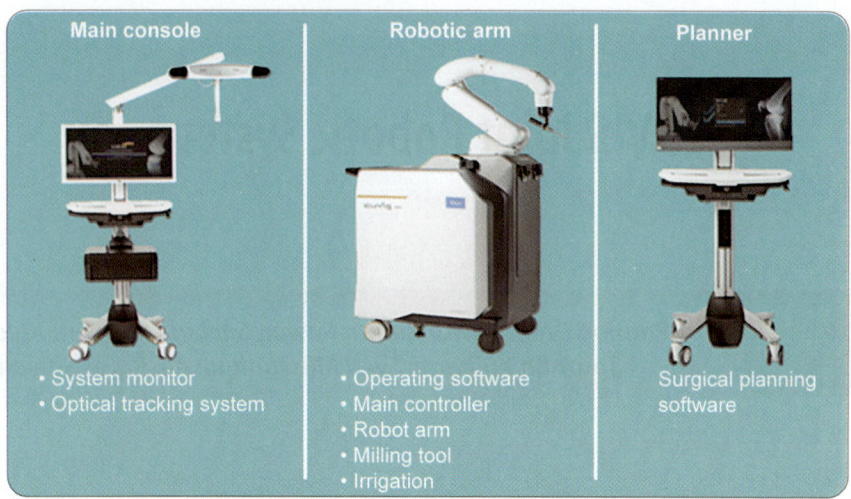

FIG. 6.1: Component of CUVIS robotic system.

with a robotic arm. The upper and lower drawers can hold operating pendants and connecting cables.
- *Dimensions*: 1,040 mm (length) × 2,340 mm (width) × 650 mm (height).
- *Weight*: 78 kg

Robotic Arm

Consists of a base, manipulator, and various peripherals, the main component used to cut the affected part by mounting a cutting tool assembly at the tip of the manipulator.
- *Dimensions*: 602 mm (length) × 648.5 mm (width) × 1,072 mm (height)
- *Weight*: 266 kg

The robotic arm of CUVIS has a 6-axis design for precise maneuverability **(Fig. 6.2)**. Six-axis design has 6 joints through which the robot can articulate to achieve fine movements. This 6-axis design provides flexibility to reach complex angles during surgery and enables accurate tool positioning of cutting tools. This robotic arm has positional accuracy of <1 mm and <1°. It also has repetition of cut, accuracy of ±0.5 mm.

The cutting motor **(Fig. 6.3)** drive is mounted on the end-effector of the robotic arm to cut the patient's bones. Since a plastic bracket exists between the pre-end of the manipulator and the tool changer, the cutting tool, including the tool changer, is electrically insulated from the manipulator. The applied part is defined as a cutter on the cutting tool assembly. Therefore, the mounting is electrically separated, so surgical cutting tools are treated as type B.

Panel Console

Equipped with a panel console (PC) that is equipped with surgery planning software, jPlanner, and installed in the operating room (OR), when a detailed surgery plan change function is required during surgery.

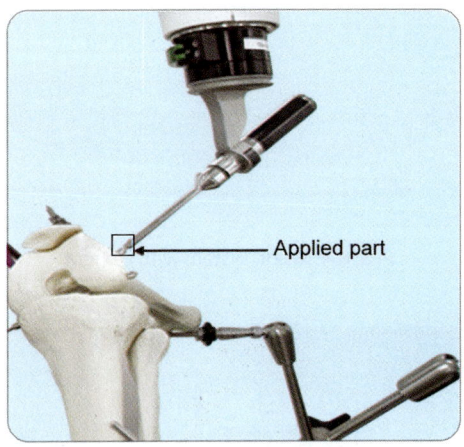

FIG. 6.2: Robotic arm.

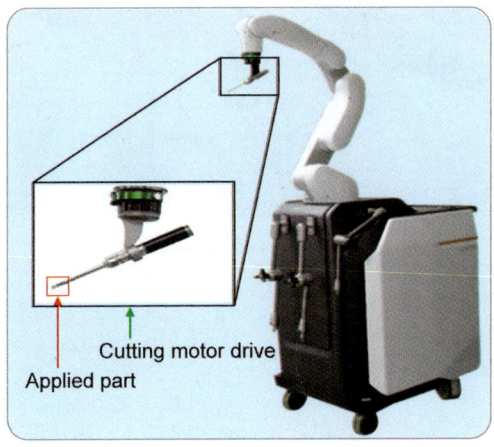

FIG. 6.3: Main console.

Vision System and Marker Specifications

It is a camera of the OTS, which is used to recognize the location of the robotic arm and the affected part of the patient **(Fig. 6.4)**.

This system uses passive tracker balls. Four such reflective trackballs make one marker. There are five such markers used. Tibial marker, femoral marker, probe marker, robot base marker, and robot arm marker **(Fig. 6.5)**.

Margin of error of this tracking system is only ± 0.2 mm **(Figs. 6.6A and B)**.

The minimum distance required for capturing of these trackers is 950 mm. Hence, the cart should be a minimum of 1 m away from the table.

CUVIS Preplanner Software

- As CUVIS is an image-based system, it requires a CT scan for preplanning. A CT scan should be done from the femoral head to the ankle.

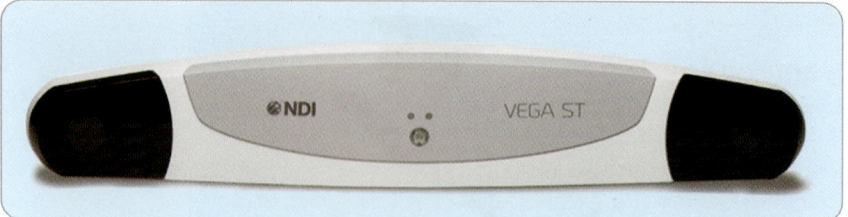

FIG. 6.4: Vision system with camera.

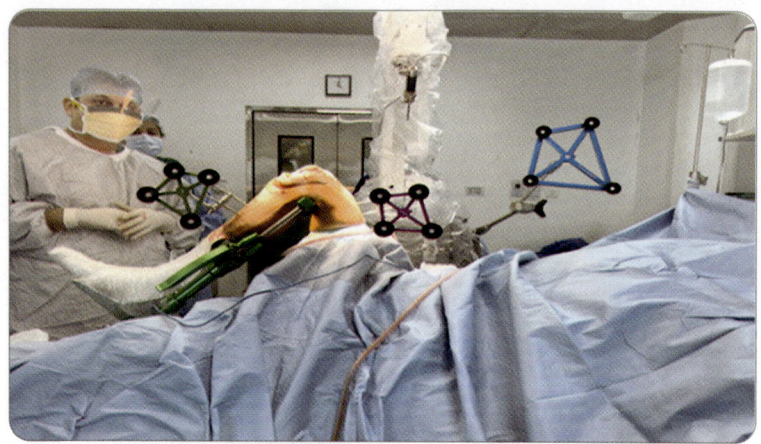

FIG. 6.5: Markers of the vision system.

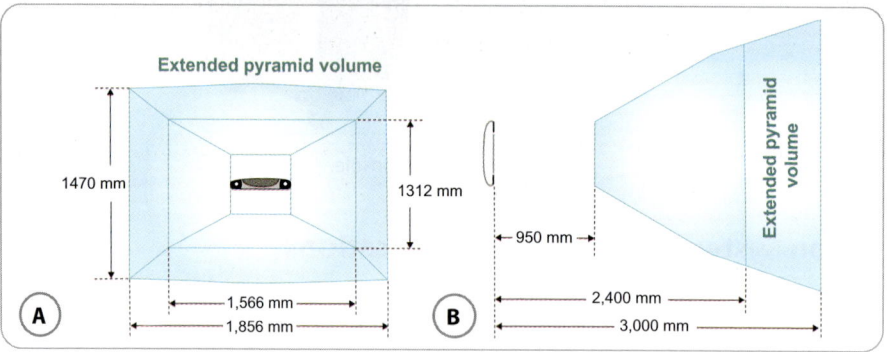

FIGS. 6.6A AND B: Area required by the tracking system.

- *CT requirements*: It is necessary to keep a metal rod near the lower limb while performing a CT scan. The purpose of this rod is stabilization of the leg and to act as a reference for processing CT images in software.
    - Matrix size 512 × 512 or 768 × 768
    - Slice thickness 1 mm or 1.25 mm
    - Number of images: 500–700
    - Voltage 120 kV, current 200 mA

Environmental Requirements

Operating Conditions
- Temperature 10–30°C
- Relative humidity 30–70% (noncondensing)
- Atmospheric pressure 700–1,060 hPa

Storage Conditions
- Temperature 0–40°C
- Relative humidity 10–90% (noncondensing)
- Atmospheric pressure 700–1,060 hPa

Electrical Specification
- *Voltage*: Single phase AC 100–240 V
- *Frequency* 50–60 Hz
- *Power consumption*:
  - Main console 0.5 kVA
  - Robotic arm 1.0 kVA
  - Planner console 0.5 kVA

PROCEDURE

Computed Tomography Scan

All surgical patients require a CT scan of the operating limb in three axial planes: The hip region, knee joints, and ankle. The 3D model derived from CT-scan images gives the operating surgeon a submillimeter accuracy for planning of precise bone resection, implant sizing, and positioning **(Fig. 6.7)**.

Surgical Planning

Preoperative surgical planning is of utmost importance as it provides the surgeon with complete surgical simulation for precise execution of the procedure

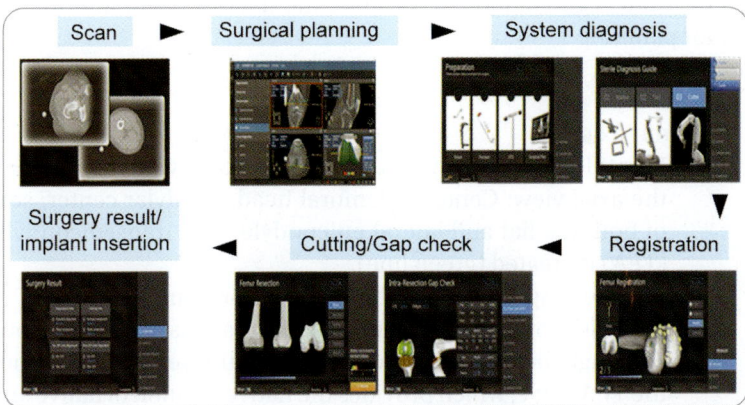

FIG. 6.7: Procedure of TKR using CUVIS system.

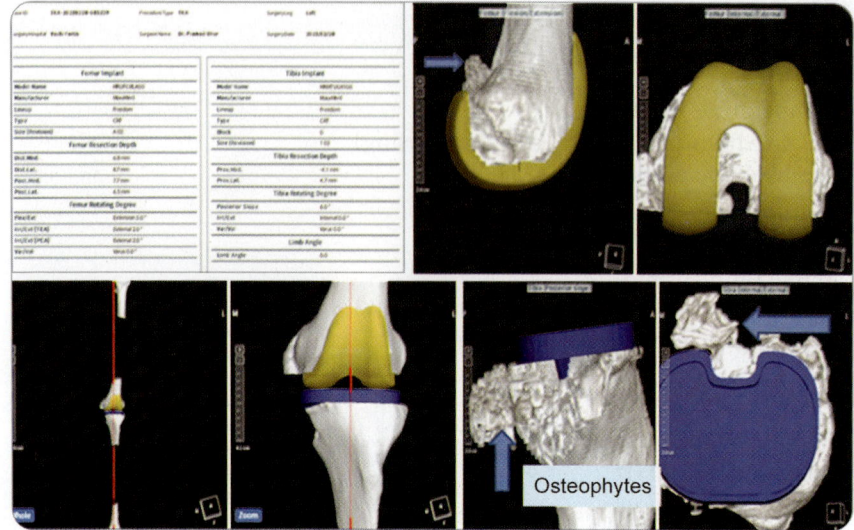

FIG. 6.8: The process of surgical planning.

(Fig. 6.8). To avoid complications like femoral notching, medial-lateral shift of implant, good preoperative planning is required.

Steps Involved in Surgical Planning
- *Uploading DICOM files*: The CT scan images are retrieved and sent to the J-Planer for segmentation in order to accomplish spatial matches with the patient's leg and the three-dimensional structure utilized in the operating SW (jSUI). A trained company employee and operating surgeon performed the planning, after which the surgical plan was saved.
- *Auto segmentation*: The artificial intelligence process of the robot will plan using software to differentiate and map the bony areas of the hip, knee, and ankle area. The process is fully automatic and takes around 15 minutes to get bone segmentation, which is started by the mechanical axis of the femur. Once the auto segmentation is finished, the data is saved, and the result is ready for planning.
- *Final planning*:
  - Femur:
    - Femur axis:
      - Identification of bony landmarks in coronal view, the sagittal view, the axial view: Center of femoral head, condylar center, selection of both medial and lateral epicondyle—the transepicondylar axis (TEA) is created (green line).
      - By selecting both the lateral posterior condyle and the medial posterior condyle, a posterior condylar axis is created (yellow line).
      - The angle between the green line and the yellow line is known as the TEA angle, which provides the native rotation of native anatomy **(Fig. 6.9)**.

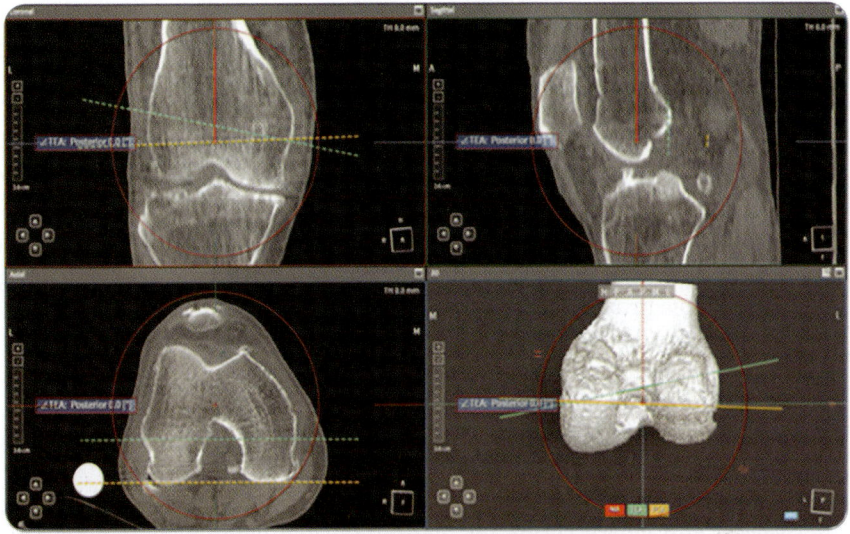

FIG. 6.9: Transepicondylar axis (TEA) angle.

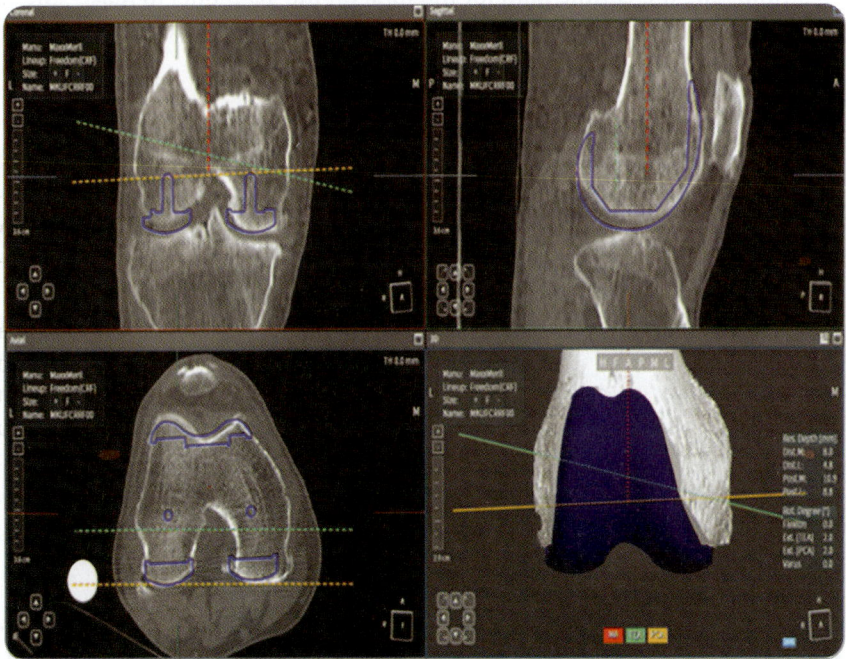

FIG. 6.10: Femur implant position.

- *Femur implant positioning (Fig. 6.10)*: After we set the mechanical axis of the Femur, the implant setting screen is populated. We have various options of flexion/extension, Internal/external, varus/valgus for optimization of the coverage and fit of the implant on the 3D bone model.

- *Femur registration points*—set on a 3D bone model to be marked on the femur are: Medial, lateral, distal, anterior medial, anterior lateral, posterior medial, and posterior lateral.
  - Tibia:
    - *Tibia axis*: Tibia mechanical axis proximal center, ankle center, tibial tuberosity, PCL fossa center, medial condyle center, lateral condyle center.
    - *Tibia implant positioning* **(Fig. 6.11)**: Next, we set the resection depth column. With the help of rotation keys, we can set the following things:
      - Tibia proximal cuts
      - Slope degree selections
      - Varus and valgus angulations
      - Internal and external rotations of the tibia
- Then we select the size of the tibial base plate depending on the following points:
  - Anterior sitting
  - Posterior sitting
  - Medial and lateral sitting for planning of reduction osteotomy in some cases
  - Native posterior slope versus tibial slope
  - Adjusting the cutting path for the tibia on the 3D model to make sure the milling device does not reach the soft tissues in the posterior, medial, and lateral aspects of the tibia
  - *Rotation keys*:
    - Tibial registration points: In all four views, i.e., the coronal view, the sagittal view, the axial view, and the 3D bone view, we have to choose six registration points that have to be reproduced in the operating

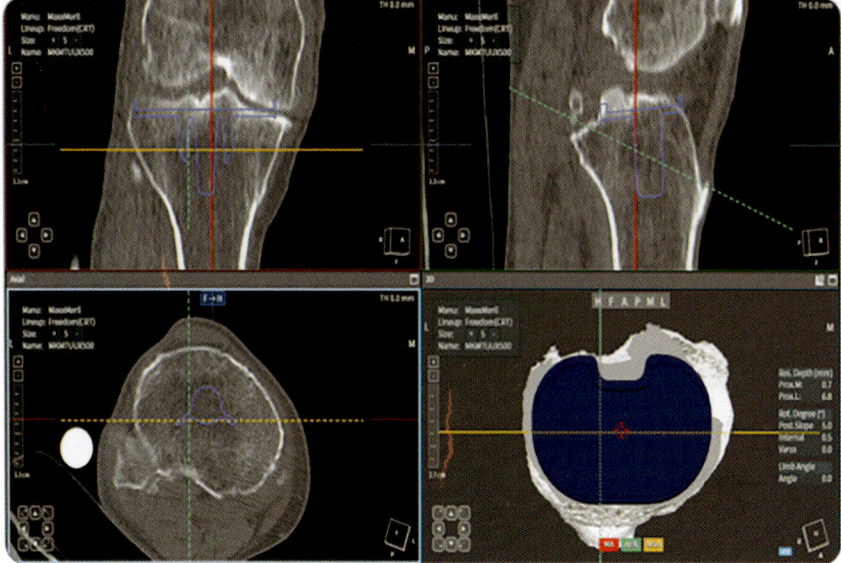

FIG. 6.11: Tibial implant position.

theatre. These points are medial, lateral, anterior, tibial tuberosity, medial plateau, and lateral plateau.
- *Final plan*: An important factor deciding implant size and flexion extension of the implant in preoperative planning is the posterior condylar cut **(Fig. 6.12)**. Recommended posterior condylar cut values for Meril implant (freedom and opulent knee) are as follows.

Freedom knee: Post condylar bone resection (mm)
- Usually, in varus deformity cut is matched with the posterolateral cut, and in valgus deformity cut is matched with the posteromedial.
- After all the marking, we get the final plan **(Figs. 6.13A to C)** and save which is later approved and downloaded.

A	B	C	D	E	F	G	H
7.2	7.7	8.2	8.5	8.8	9.4	9.8	10.4

FIG. 6.12: Recommended posterior condyle cuts.

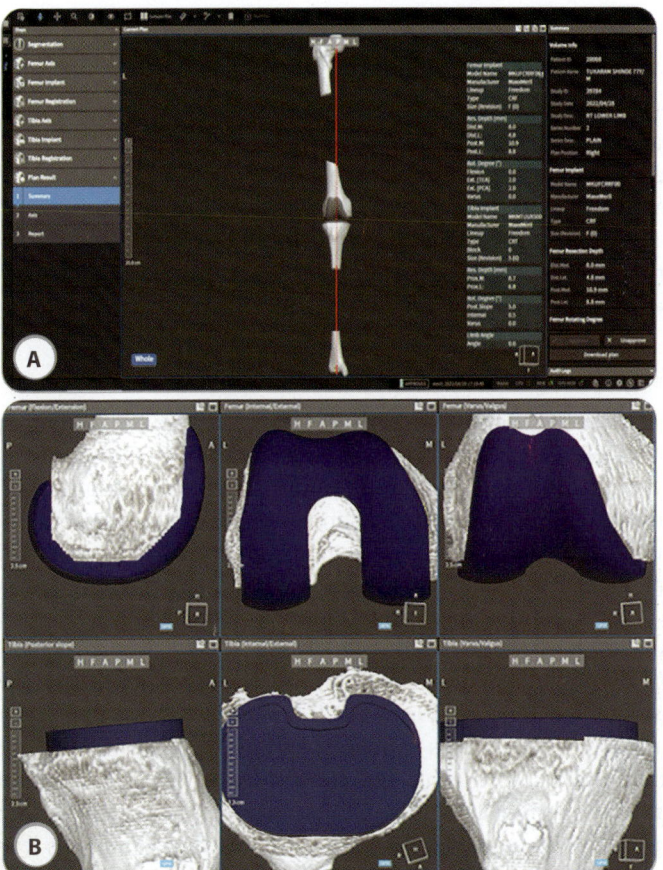

FIGS. 6.13A TO C: *Continued*

Continued

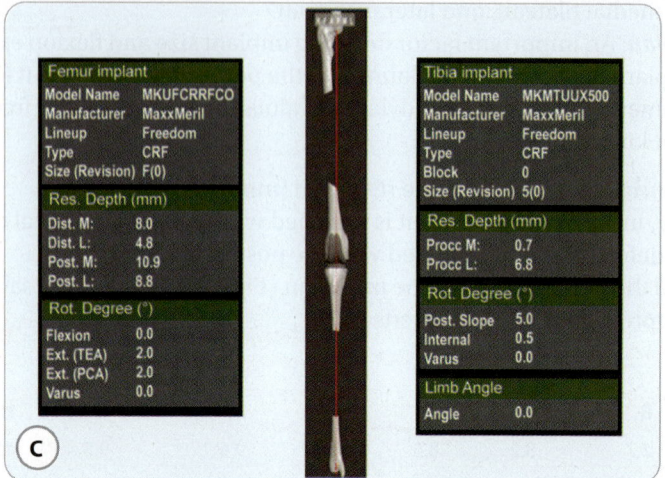

FIGS. 6.13A TO C: (A) Final; (B) Final 3D model of knee with implant; and (C) Final 3D model of knee with resection depth.

System Diagnosis

- This procedure is done in the operating theatre at the time of patient preparation.
- "Marker," "Tool," "Cutter" step-by-step.
- "Marker" stage assembles and checks multiple instruments.
- "Tool" step performs verification of the robotic arm for surgery.
- "Cutter" stage checks the cutter tool for surgery.
- After each step is completed, you can proceed to the next step.

Registration

Knee joint exposure is done as per standard protocols of the operating surgeon. Arthrotomy is performed, menisci are excised, and in the following step, the surgeon inserts the femur marker over the unicortical Schanz pin of 4 mm diameter and length of 160 mm in the same incision over the anteromedial cortex of the femur. For the tibia marker, a small incision is made 10–15 cm distal to the joint line, and a unicortical Schanz screw of 140 mm length is inserted across the drill guide in the anteromedial cortex **(Figs. 6.14A to D)**.

Surgeons then determine the marker's position depending on the OTS camera, and then set the marker's direction so that these marker arrays are visible in both flexion and extension **(Fig. 6.15)**.

The surgeon then performs spatial matching between the patient's leg and the 3D model utilized in the surgical plan **(Fig. 6.16)**. This is done by surface registration of the femur and tibia using a probe. Subsequently, the computer generates a virtual 3D image of the knee, and the system matches it with the CT images. The registration needs to be precise, which is indicated by a final root mean square (RMS) error of <1.

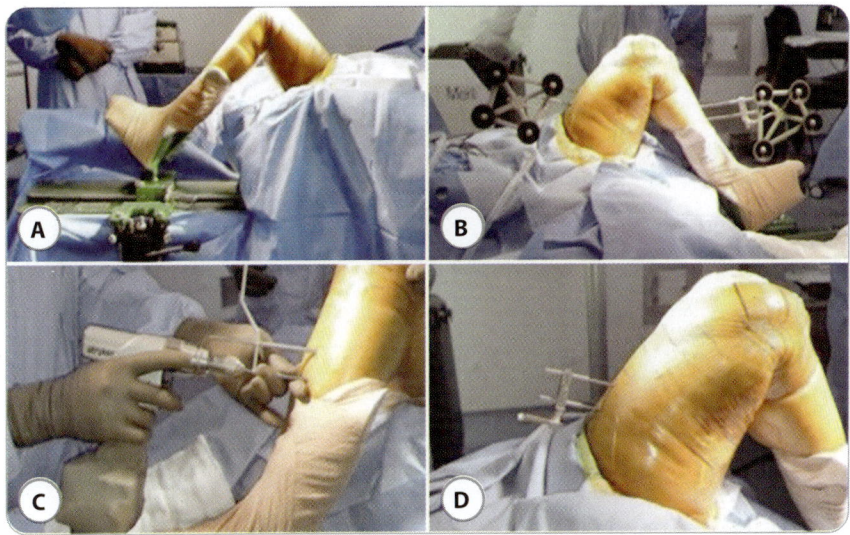

FIGS. 6.14A TO D: Pin placement for the markers.

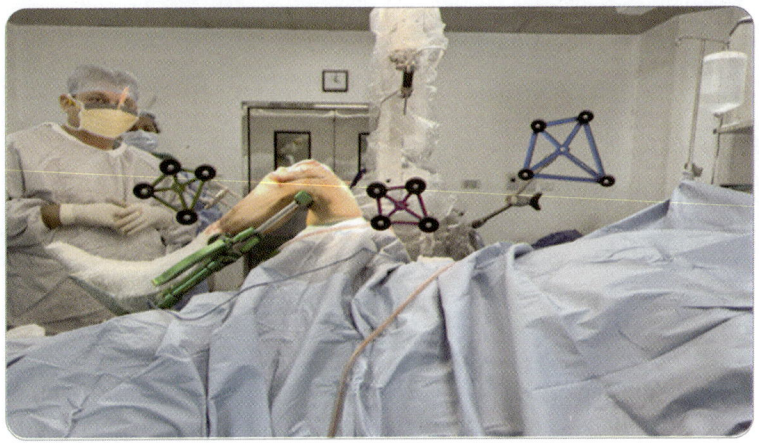

FIG. 6.15: Markers of the vision system.

Now, 40 points are needed to be collected over the femur in six groups (distal medial, trochlear, distal lateral, medial notch, lateral notch, medial cortex and anterior), and 40 points must be gained over the tibia in six groups (proximal medial, tibial spine, proximal lateral, medial, tibial tuberosity and anterior) **(Figs. 6.17A and B)**.

Gap Check

At this point, the role of the surgeon is important; it is the surgeon who decides the alignment method to be used for the case. After the registration process of both femur and tibia is complete, pre-resection (before robotic cutting), a gap check is performed. In this step, mechanical alignment or restricted kinematic alignment,

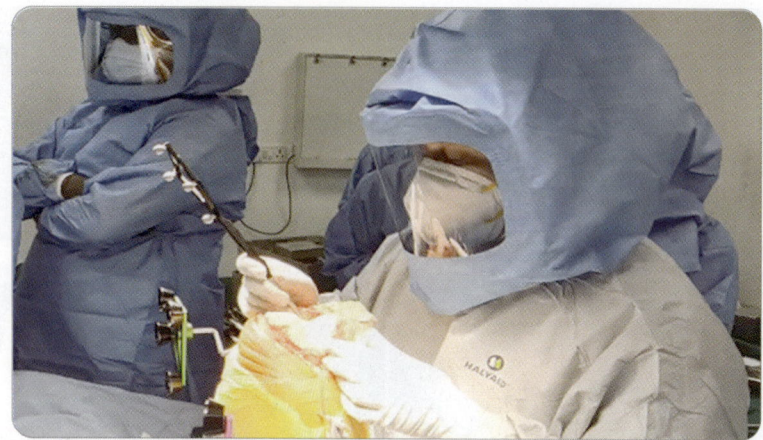

FIG. 6.16: Surgeon doing surface registration and as seen on the screen.

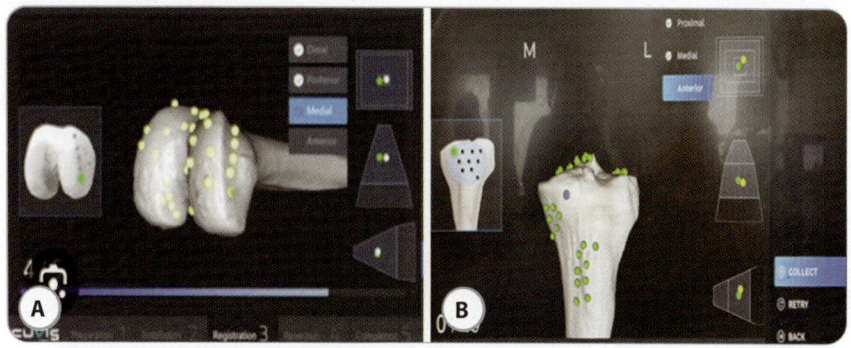

FIGS. 6.17A AND B: Points collection on femur and tibia.

or kinematic alignment principles can be applied as per the surgeon's preference. Surgeons have to balance medial and lateral gaps in extension and flexion (90°). Depending upon the volume of osteophytes difference of 1–3 mm between medial and lateral gaps is considered a balanced joint **(Figs. 6.18A and B)**.

If osteophytes are already removed, then gap balancing values equal on both sides (9 mm) are acceptable. And this is achieved by adjusting implant positioning. Methodology for correcting gap imbalance by adjusting implant positioning is given below **(Table 6.1)**.

Cutting

After the gap balancing is achieved, the knee is fixed in flexion of 115°. As this is an active, autonomous cutting system, no bone movements are acceptable during bone cutting. To prevent such bone movement, knee positioner (to hold leg in flexed position) and bone clamps or femoral/tibial pins (for bone holding) are used during the surgery **(Fig. 6.19)**.

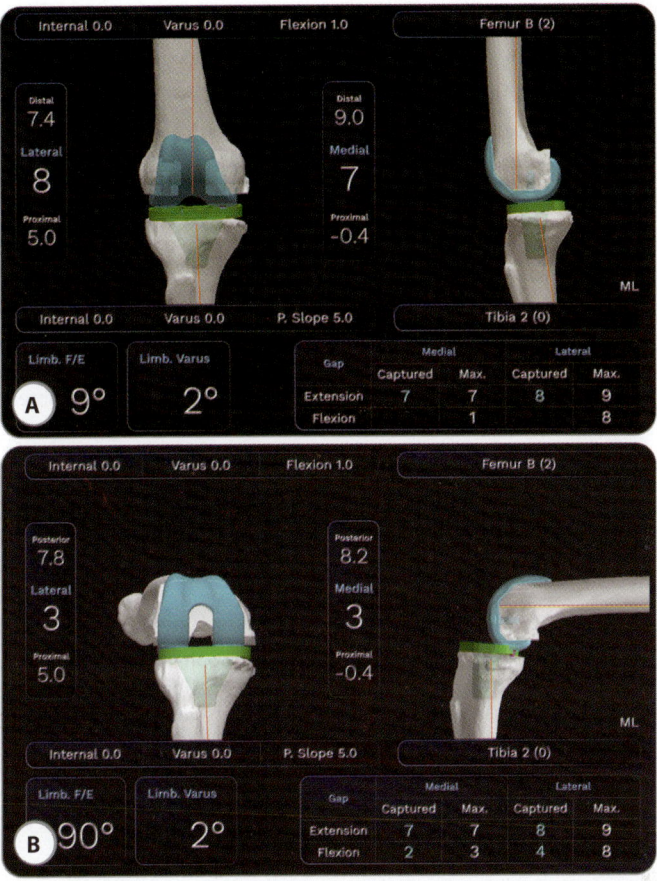

FIGS. 6.18A AND B: (A) Pre-resection extension gap check; and (B) Pre-resection flexion gap check.

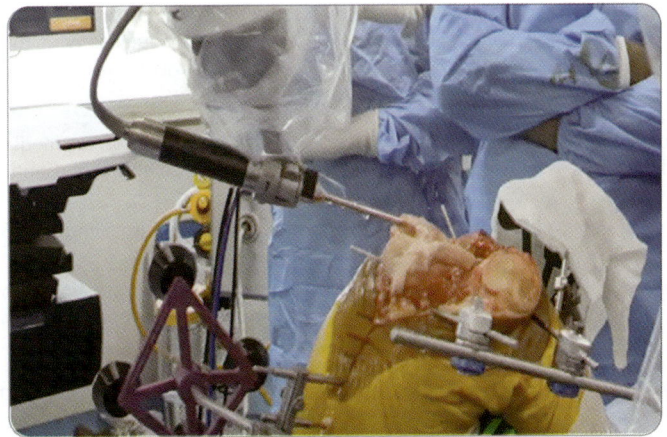

FIG. 6.19: Femoral pins to mount the robot.

TABLE 6.1: The technique of gap balancing.

Intraoperative scenario	Adjustments
Excess gap in both flexion and extension	Proximalize the tibial component
Decreased gap in both flexion and extension	Distalize the tibial component
Balanced extension, tight flexion	• Downsize the femoral component (anterior referencing). Posterior condylar offset ratio (Posterior condylar offset/femoral diameter) is maintained < 95% • Shift the femoral component anteriorly but limit it to 2 mm to avoid overstuffing of the patellofemoral joint. The anterior femoral offset is maintained < 15% • Adjust the posterior slope of the tibia maximum up to 7° • Shift the tibial component distally, resulting in an increase in both flexion and extension gaps, hence to be followed by distalizing the femoral component to balance the extension gap
Balanced extension, lax flexion	• Posteriorize (max 1 mm) and flex (maximum 2°) the femoral component to decrease the flexion gap. Avoid anterior notching with careful visualization clinically and using robot monitors • Proximalization of the tibial component, which decreases both extension-flexion gaps hence to be followed by proximalization of the femoral component to increase the extension gaps
Balanced flexion, lax extension	Distalize the femoral component
Balanced flexion, tight extension	Proximalize the femoral component
Tight medial gaps in flexion and extension	*Consideration*: Check for posteromedial osteophytes in the femur and tibia on the X-rays, and if present, anticipate laxity after osteophyte removal • Place the tibial component in varus (maximum 4°) • Perform soft tissue releases in the following order: Deep medial collateral ligament (MCL), posterior oblique ligament, medial reduction osteotomy, semimembranosus release, pie crusting of the superficial MCL
Balanced extension, tight medial flexion gap	*Consideration*: Check for posterior osteophytes on the medial femoral condyles. If present, leave the medial space untouched, anticipating laxity after osteophyte removal. If absent: • Externally rotate the femoral component (maximum 3° to the surgical TEA) • Perform soft tissue release medially and pie crusting of the anterior MCL fibers. It is important to note that osteophyte removal can increase both flexion and extension gaps
Balanced flexion, tight medial extension gap	Place the femoral component in varus (maximum 3°) and further perform soft tissue release if needed. Based on the gaps, the femoral component is placed within 3° of valgus to 3° of varus
Tibial posterior slope	Based on the preoperative CT measurements, adjust the posterior slope up to a maximum of 7° to increase the flexion gap

The robot is fastened to a patient and stabilized near the operating table as per the instructions. The robot cart is on the ipsilateral side, and the vision cart is placed on the opposite side. **Figures 6.20A and B** show the position of the robot in OR and the surgeon.

The guide on this screen indicates the present surface of the femur to be sliced and aids a total of six cutting planes **(Fig. 6.21)**. The operating software (jSUI) enables the surgical robot to cut the bone at an exact angle and orientation.

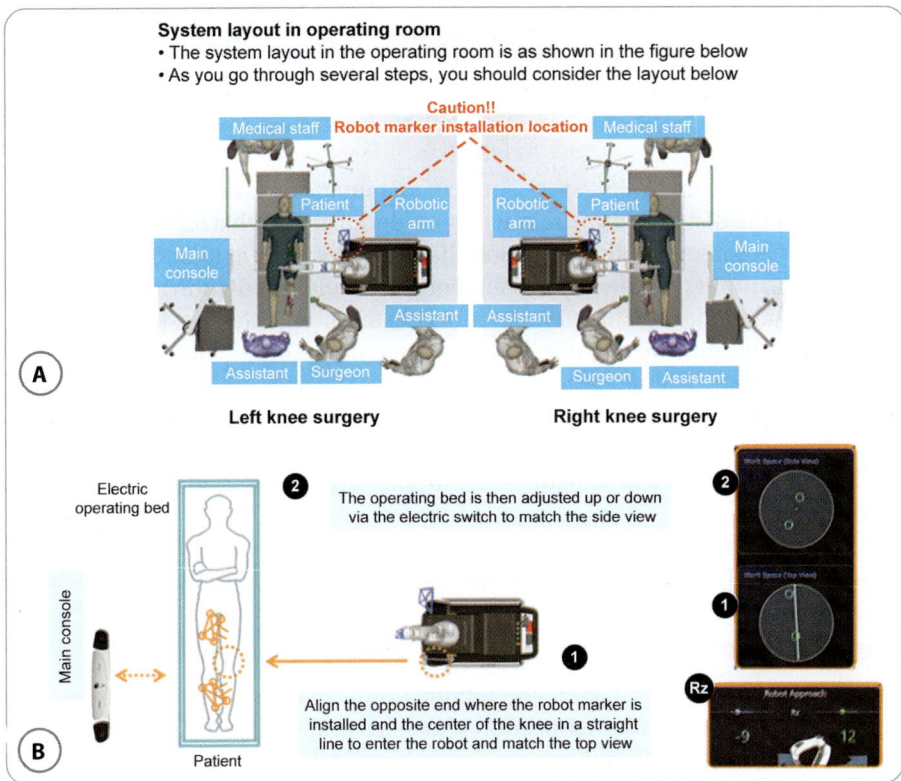

FIGS. 6.20A AND B: (A) System layout in operating room (OR); and (B) Position of the robot and main console in OR.

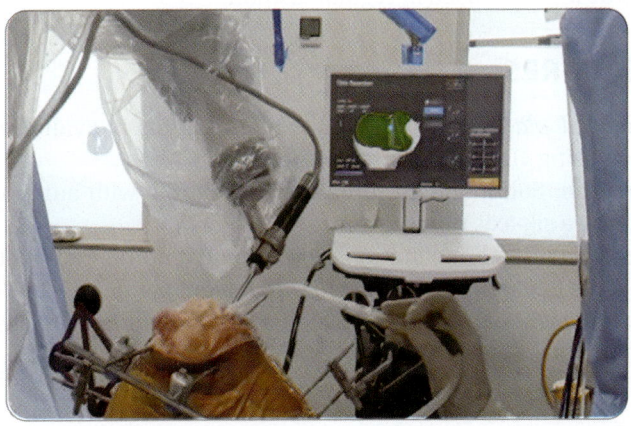

FIG. 6.21: Resection done by robotic arm.

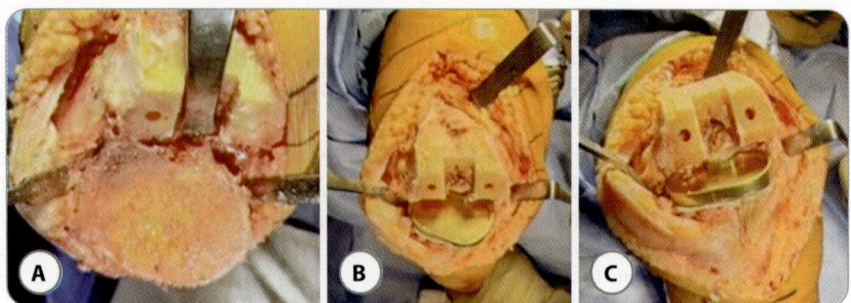

FIGS. 6.22A TO C: Postresection of the femur and tibia.

The robotic arm mills each surface systematically, beginning with the resection of the distal femur. The resection is performed with a 6.2 mm burr with continuous automated saline irrigation that mills the bone at a predefined level, based on the input provided by the surgeon. The femur is cut individually, in the order of distal, anterior chamfer, anterior, posterior chamfer, posterior, and so on. Tibia is cut individually, one face at a time, in the order "medial" and then "lateral." The type of bone resection is decided by the operating surgeon; it could be either extension surface resection or full surface resection. **Figure 6.22** shows the postresection bony surface of the femur and tibia.

The advantage of this system is that it also prepares the tibial keel with a robotic arm.

With restricted bone cutting and advanced features like bone movement monitoring (BMM), CUVIS joint offers maximum safety to the surgeons.

Implant Insertion

Once all the cuts are completed, the robotic arm is manually detached from the patient's body, and standard procedures such as removal of the remaining bone islands, removal of posterior osteophytes, and menisci are performed as required. The ligament balance is checked **(Figs. 6.23A and B)** and documented after inserting trial implants after this assessment final implant is inserted **(Figs. 6.24A and B)**, and the knee is closed in regular fashion.

KEY FEATURES

- *Individualized planning*: Preoperative planning for individualized implant placement using 3D CT and virtual simulation.
- *High precision*: Submillimeter precision is possible with autonomous bone cutting using a six-axis robotic arm.
- *Real-time safety*: The bone motion monitor and a number of safety measures (such as force freeze and emergency stop) ensure patient safety.
- *Advanced navigation*: A sophisticated OTS that offers precise, real-time surgical guidance.

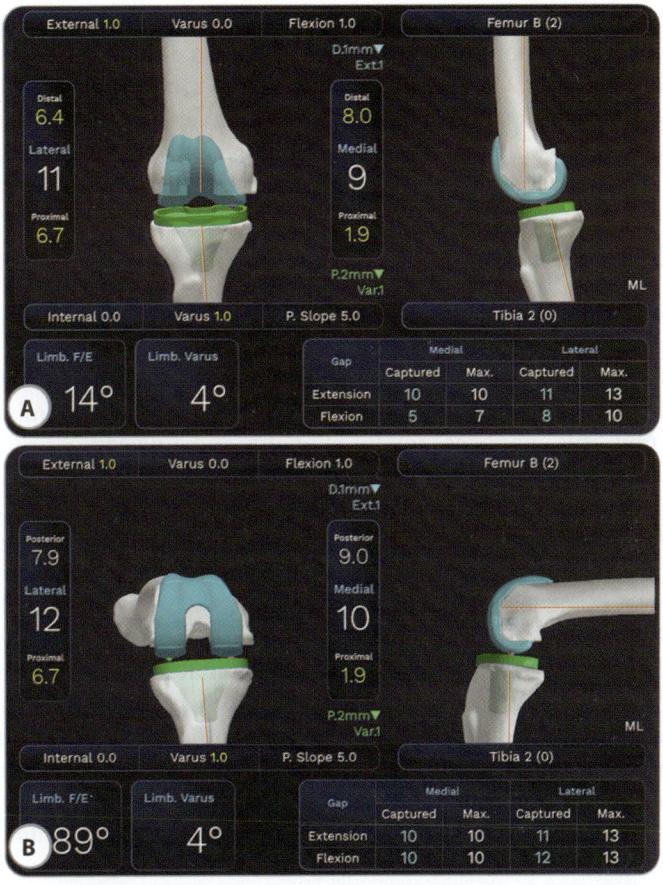

FIGS. 6.23A AND B: (A) Postresection extension gap check; and (B) Postresection flexion gap check.

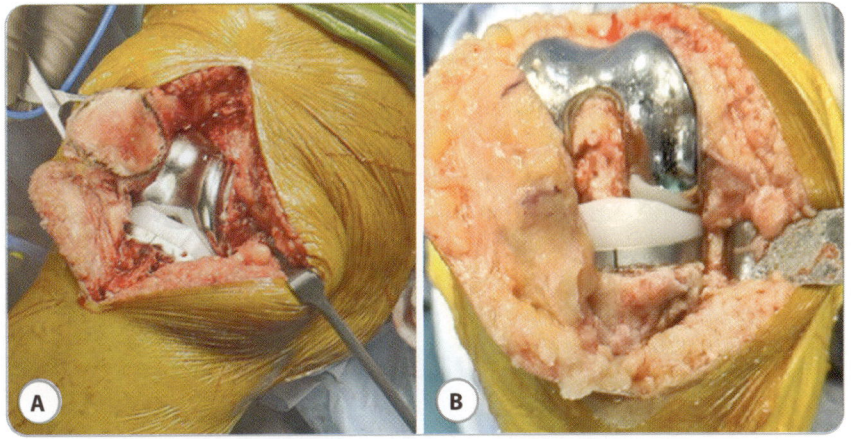

FIGS. 6.24A AND B: Final implants placed.

- *Flexible execution*: Enables intraoperative adjustments and complete or partial incisions for optimal outcomes.
- *Minimally invasive*: Compared to conventional procedures, it reduces blood loss and shortens hospital stays and recovery times.
- *User-friendly*: A compact design and intuitive software simplify the surgical procedure.

CONCLUSION

With its unmatched precision, safety, and customization, the CUVIS Joint Robotic System is a major advancement in TKR surgery.

The system guarantees the best possible implant placement and alignment by utilising 3D preplanning, real-time intraoperative adjustments, and automated precise cutting. This enhances joint functionality and longevity.

Its dependability is highlighted by studies that show its safety with no notable intraoperative complications, including an analysis of 500 cases in India.

The system is a revolutionary tool for treating complicated knee conditions like osteoarthritis and deformities because of its capacity to minimize tissue damage, lower blood loss, and speed up recovery.

The CUVIS system reduces the risk of complications like limb length inequality and fractures by providing better femoral and tibial alignment accuracy than traditional TKR.

Being a completely self-sufficient robotic platform, it enables surgeons to produce reliable, consistent results, enhancing patient happiness and quality of life. The CUVIS Joint Robotic System is a ground-breaking advancement in orthopedic surgery that is raising the bar for accuracy and patient-focused treatment.

CHAPTER 7

MISSO Robotic System

Sourabh Kulkarni, Pramod Bhor, Sachin Yashwant Kale

INTRODUCTION

The MISSO Robotic system is a fully active surgical robot developed in India by Meril Healthcare Pvt Ltd This system integrates real-time intraoperative feedback with submillimeter precision and personalized preoperative planning to optimize implant alignment. It is equipped with a 6-axis articulated robotic arm, advanced imaging capabilities, and a host of safety features, including bone movement monitoring and emergency stop mechanisms **(Fig. 7.1)**.

Moreover, the cost-effective nature of a domestically produced system is its beneficial aspect. MISSO has been developed with local anatomical and clinical challenges in mind, such as the higher prevalence of osteoporosis and unique joint degeneration patterns in Indian patients.

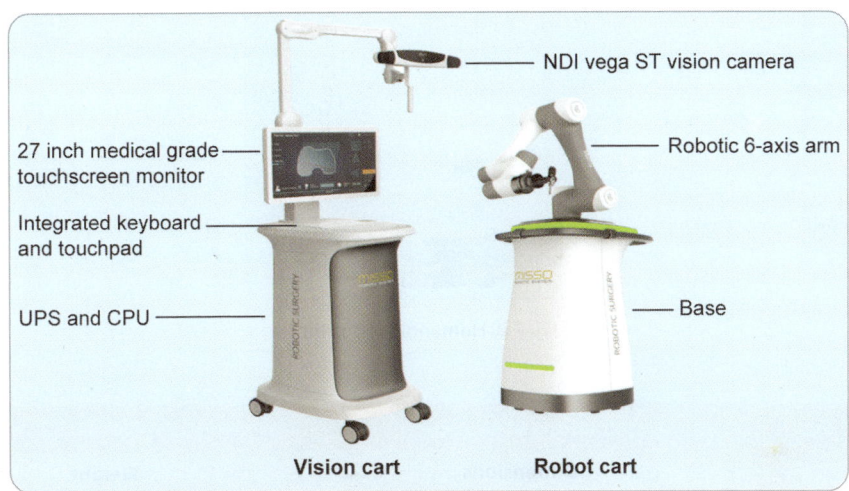

FIG. 7.1: MISSO robotic system.

ROBOT DIMENSIONS AND WEIGHT

Shape and Ergonomic Design

Amongst all floor-mounted robots, MISSO has the smallest footprint **(Fig. 7.2)**. The advantage of this is being the least imposing robot to work with **(Table 7.1)**. Storage and maneuverability are easier.

ROBOTIC ARM SPECIFICATIONS

The robotic arm of MISSO has a 6-axis design for precise maneuverability. Six-Axis design has six joints through which the robot can articulate to achieve fine movements **(Fig. 7.3)**. This 6-axis design provides flexibility to reach complex angles during surgery and enables accurate tool positioning of the cutting tool. This robotic arm has positional accuracy of <1 mm and <1°. It also has repetition of cut, accuracy of ±0.5 mm. J2 has a 160° range of motion. Rest all other five joints (J1, J3, J4, J5, and J6) have 360° maneuverability. The working radius of this arm is 900 mm (35.4 in).

VISION SYSTEM AND MARKER SPECIFICATIONS

Network device interface (NDI) camera works on the principle of infrared light. NDI camera has both an infrared light transmitter and receiver **(Fig. 7.4)**. The infrared light reflected from a specifically designed marker is captured in the

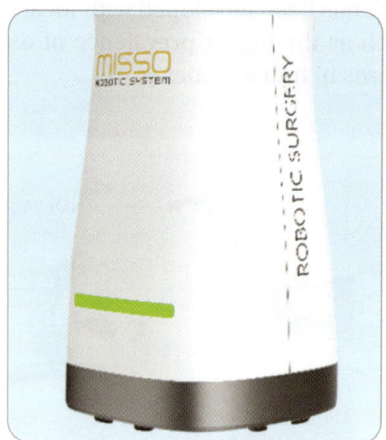

FIG. 7.2: Humanoid footprint.

TABLE 7.1: Design specifications of MISSO.		
	Dimensions	Weight
MISSO robot cart	560 mm (W) × 700 mm (D) × 1600 mm (H)	170 kg
MISSO vision cart	660 mm (W) × 700 mm (D) × 2,200 mm (H)	210 kg

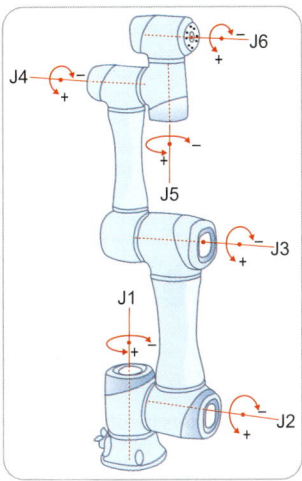

FIG. 7.3: Six-axis design.

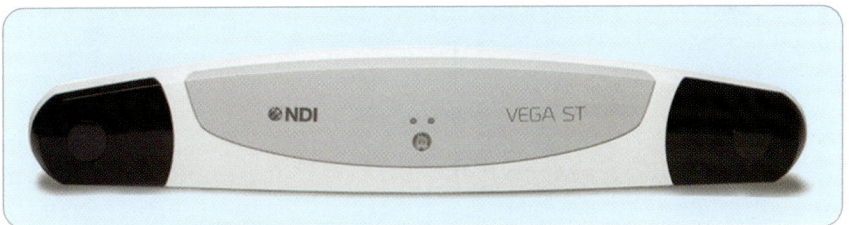

FIG. 7.4: Network device interface camera.

camera. Such markers have a high reflectivity index. The spherical shape of these markers makes them easier to identify at various angles. The markers are combined in a plane in a unique configuration that helps to define a plane. Markers arranged in a plane are then further used to track the rigid body motion of the objects under consideration. Hence, the entire system, including the camera and markers, is called the optical tracking system.

Two types of markers are used in the optical tracking system: Passive and active. Passive markers need an infrared light source from the camera. The light reflected from these markers is used for tracking. On the other hand, active markers have their own source of generating infrared light.

This system uses passive tracker balls. Four such reflective tracker balls make one marker. There are five such markers. Tibial marker, femoral marker, probe marker, robot base marker, and robot arm marker **(Fig. 7.5)**.

The margin of error of this tracking system is only ±0.2 mm.

The minimum distance required for capturing of these trackers is 950 mm. Hence, the cart should be a minimum of 1 m away from the table **(Fig. 7.6)**.

This system comes with a 27 inches *touchscreen medical-grade monitor*.

This robotic system is equipped with an inbuilt UPS system for uninterrupted operation in situations of power failure. One leg's entire surgery can be performed on UPS power under standard conditions.

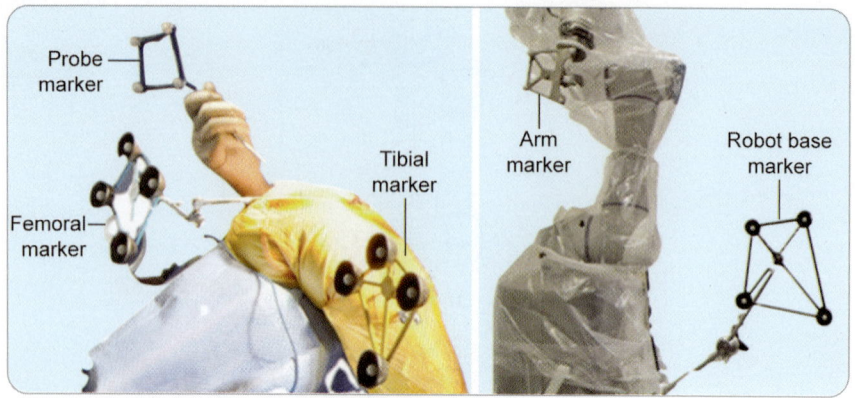

FIG. 7.5: Markers in robotic surgery.

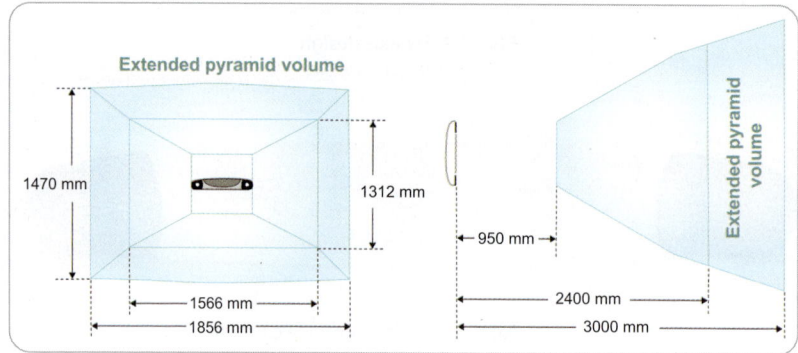

FIG. 7.6: Camera vision.

CUTTING TOOLS AND CHUCK SYSTEM

Cutting tools have the following components **(Fig. 7.7)**:
- Cutting tool chuck
- Cutting tool sleeve (regular and short)
- High-speed cutting motor
- Bone cutter blade
- Irrigation sleeve for debris management

The high-speed cutting motor has a maximum speed of up to 70,000 RPM. Routinely 65,000 RPM speed is utilized for surgical bone cutting. Heat generated with this high-speed burr cutting is neutralized by an active irrigation system which irrigates water with adjustable speed.

Bone cutting diameter with this burr system is 6.2 mm. This burr blade is officially rated for 10 procedures under standard conditions.

Chuck, sleeve, and burr blade irrigation sleeve are all autoclavable **(Box 7.1)**.

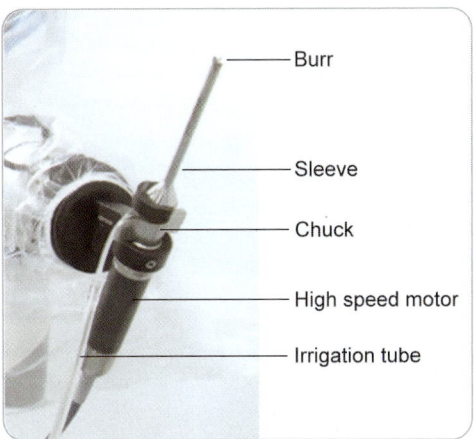

FIG. 7.7: Cutting system.

> **BOX 7.1: Computed tomography (CT) scan requirements.**
> - *Matrix size*: 512 × 512 or 768 × 768
> - *Slice thickness*: 1 or 1.25 mm
> - *Number of images*: 700–900
> - *Voltage* : 120 kV
> - *Current*: 200 mA
> - *Output*: Axial view reconstruction with single-leg focus

MISSO PREPLANNER SOFTWARE

As MISSO is an image-based system, it requires a CT scan for preplanning. A CT scan should be done from the femoral head to the ankle.

Computed Tomography Scan Requirements

It is necessary to keep a metal rod near the lower limb while performing a CT scan. This rod is provided by the robot. The purpose of this rod is stabilization of the leg and to act as a reference for processing CT images in software **(Figs. 7.8 and 7.9)**.

Planning Protocol

MISSO pre-planner software is a heavy software. Hence, a compatible laptop with high configuration is provided with the system. When CT scan data is incorporated in software, autosegmentation is done to form a three-dimensional (3D) model of the lower limb from the head of the femur to the ankle. The manual segmentation option is available.

Planning in the MISSO robotic software starts with uploading a CT scan. The CT scan is then processed, and a 3D model of the patient's leg from the femoral head center to the ankle joint is created.

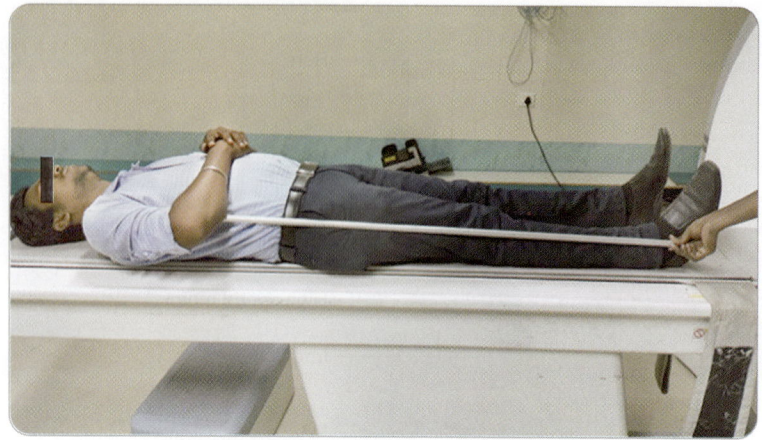

FIG. 7.8: Rod for computed tomography (CT) scan.

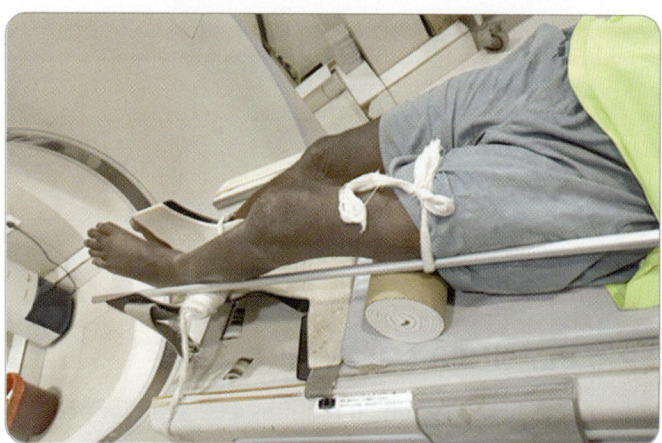

FIG. 7.9: Positioning for computed tomography (CT) scan.

This 3D model is then segmented into four segments by the process called segmentation **(Fig. 7.10)**. These four segments are: Proximal femur, distal femur, proximal tibia, and distal tibia. After segmentation, planning proceeds in six parts.

Femoral Axis

In this part seven points that define the mechanical axis of the femur are chosen. These points are the head center, femoral condyle center, medial epicondyle, lateral epicondyle, medial posterior condyle, lateral posterior condyle, medial distal condyle, and lateral distal condyle **(Box 7.2)**. These points are already chosen by the AI built into the software. But the surgeon must use his knowledge to precisely reselect these points, which in turn leads to more precision in implant placement.

Tibial Axis

After this, we must choose anatomical landmarks that define the tibial mechanical axis. These six points are the proximal center, ankle center, tibial tuberosity,

CHAPTER 7: MISSO Robotic System

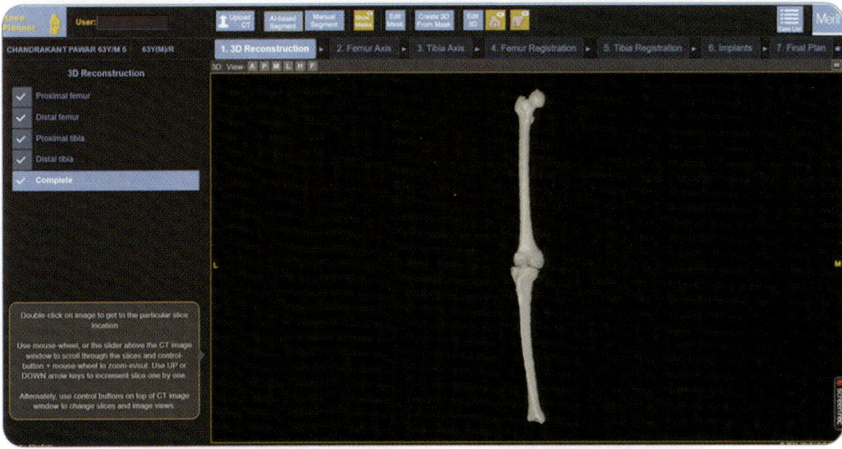

FIG. 7.10: Three-dimensional model with segmentation.

BOX 7.2: Femur axis points.

- Head center
- Condyle center
- Medial epicondyle
- Lateral epicondyle
- Medial posterior condyle
- Lateral posterior condyle
- Medial distal condyle
- Lateral distal condyle

BOX 7.3: Tibial axis points.

- Proximal center
- Ankle center
- Tuberosity
- Posterior cruciate ligament fossa center
- Medial condyle center
- Lateral condyle center

PCL fossa center, medial condyle center, and lateral condyle center **(Box 7.3)**. Similarly, these points are already chosen by AI but should be checked by an operating surgeon and reselected if necessary.

Femoral Registration

The next step is to mark femoral registration points **(Fig. 7.11)**. These are nine points that should be chosen by the operating surgeon, and these points must be reproduced in the operating theater when asked for at the time of initial mapping with precision.

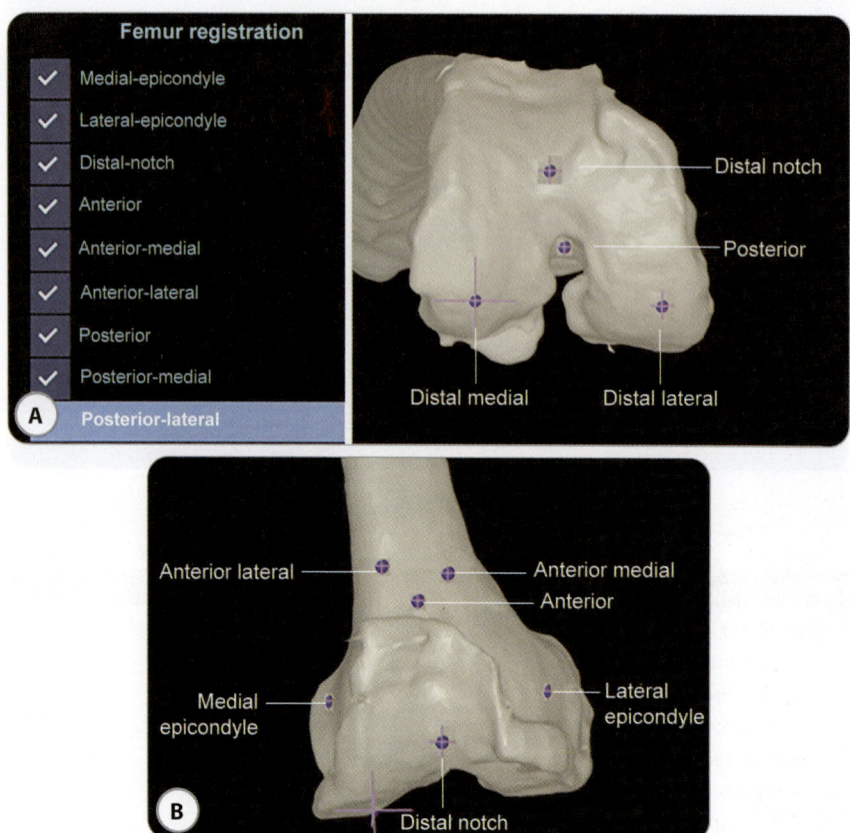

FIGS. 7.11A AND B: Femoral registration points.

Reproducing these points is important as this step defines the spatial orientation of the femur in the operating theater. This process is called initial mapping. Root mean square error (RMSE) represents the deviation of actual data given by the surgeon from CT data. Hence, the RMSE value should be smaller. Ideally RMSE initial value must be less than 10. If the initial RMSE value is >10, repetition of the initial mapping is advisable.

Tibial Registration

Similarly, seven points need to be registered for tibial registration for initial mapping **(Fig. 7.12)**. So, these points are to be chosen by the surgeon himself. As these points define the spatial orientation of the femur in the operating theater, this RMSE should also be <10.

Implant Planning

As a next step, "implant planning" is given by AI. In this implant planning process, there are four screens. The implant sitting on the bone is visualized in the coronal section, sagittal section, axial section, and 3D view orientation **(Fig. 7.13)**.

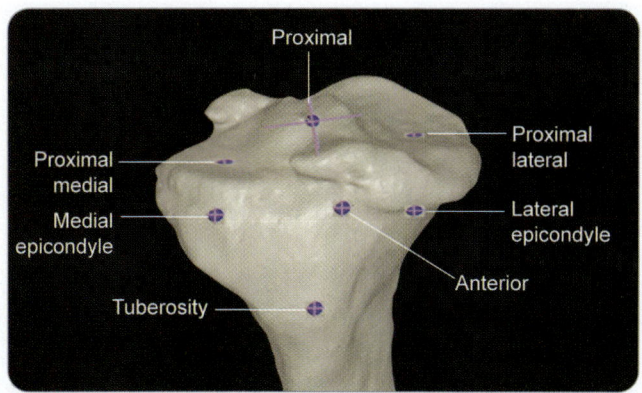

FIG. 7.12: Tibial registration points.

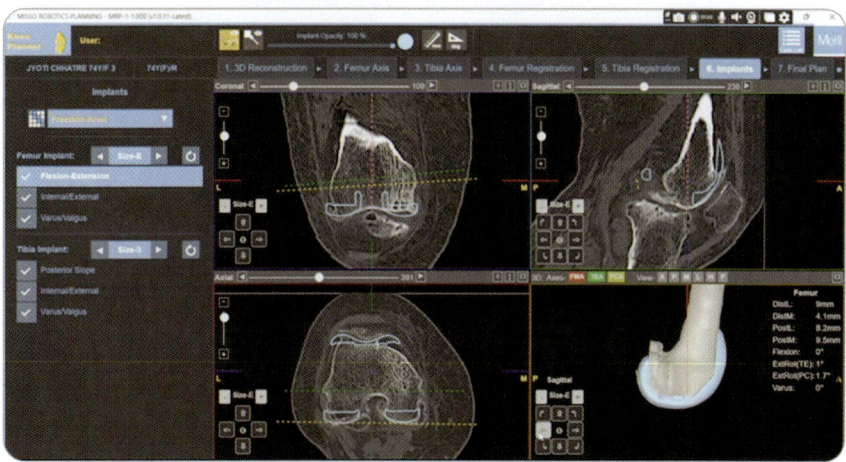

FIG. 7.13: Femoral implant planning screen.

In the coronal section medial-lateral fit of the implant has to be checked at the level of pegs **(Fig. 7.14)**. Centering the implant on the bone can be done with the help of the cursor arrows. The implant size can be changed up and down by the + and – keys.

In the axial view, two things are checked: The relationship of the implant with the native posterior condyles and the orientation of the trochlea of the implant in relationship with the patella **(Fig. 7.15)**. External or internal rotation can be done using curved cursor arrows. Also, in the sagittal view, we check the anterior notching of the femur **(Fig. 7.16)**. Then the posterior condylar fit of the implant with respect with the posterior condyles is checked. The condylar contours of the implant and native bone should match, and that usually represents the perfect replication of natural anatomy.

An important factor deciding implant size and flexion extension of the implant in preoperative planning is the posterior condylar cut. Recommended posterior condylar cut values for Meril implant (freedom and opulent knee) are as follows **(Table 7.2)**.

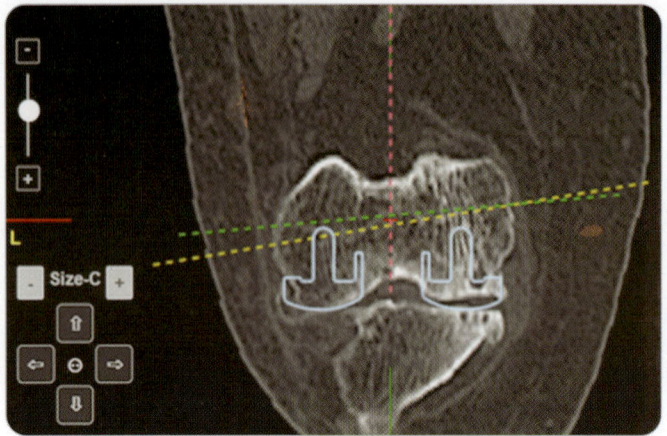

FIG. 7.14: Coronal section mesiolingual (ML) fit.

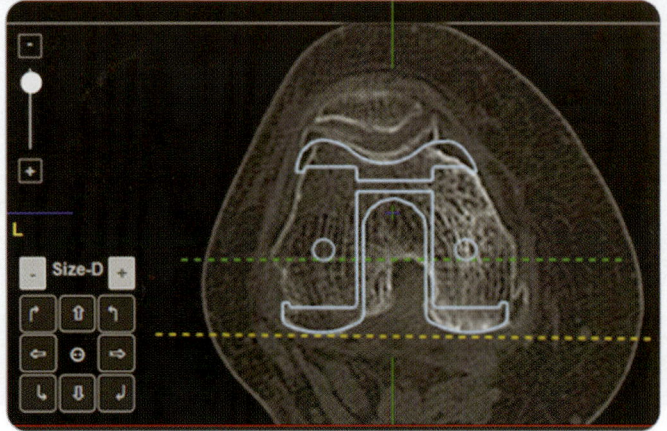

FIG. 7.15: Axial view.

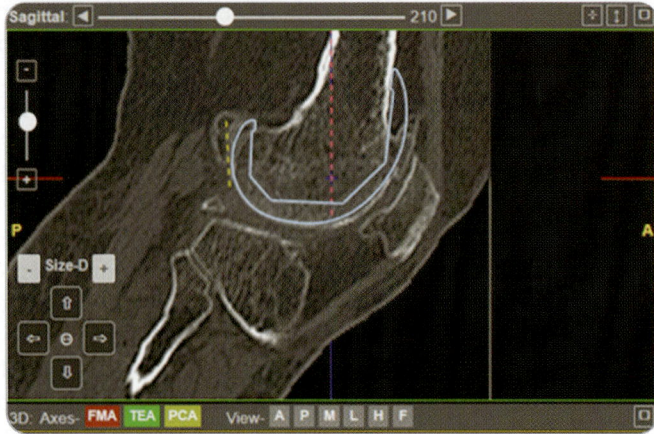

FIG. 7.16: Sagittal view.

TABLE 7.2: Posterior condylar bone resection values.

Size (mm)	A	B	C	D	E	F	G	H
	7.2	7.7	8.2	8.5	8.8	9.4	9.8	10.4

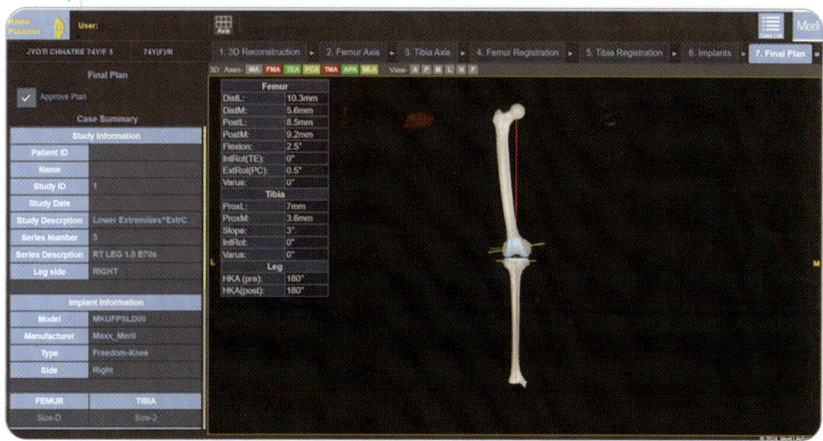

FIG. 7.17: Final plan.

Freedom Knee: Postcondylar Bone Resection (mm)

Usually, in varus deformity cut is matched with the posterolateral cut, and in valgus deformity cut is matched with the posteromedial.

Final Plan

In the last step, the final plan is given **(Fig. 7.17)**. In this plan, we can see all the cuts with their measurements, the flexion-extension of the implant, preoperative hip, knee, and ankle (HKA) axis, and postoperative HKA axis.

When a final plan is ready, it will be transferred to the robot just before the surgery. Intraoperative plan modifications can be done. Femoral size can be changed to one size up and one size down intraoperatively.

Autoclavability and Sterilization

All components, including cutting tools, marker balls, and sleeves, are autoclavable and designed for repeated sterilization cycles.

Robot Preparation before Surgery

Preparation of the robot before surgery is done while the patient is undergoing anesthesia, followed by painting and draping. This calibration process is completed in three parts: The marker test, the calibration, and the cutter test. Once these tests are satisfactorily completed, then the robotic system is ready for the surgery.

Intraoperative Protocols

The knee is exposed as per the surgeon's preference. Tibial and femoral pins (4 mm diameter) are put in with the help of a sleeve.

Tibial pins are put three to four fingerbreadths down the tibial tuberosity on an anteromedial surface.

Femoral pins can be put percutaneously through the quadriceps or can also be put anteromedially in the distal femur through an exposed knee **(Fig. 7.18)**.

Femoral and tibial markers are then fixed on corresponding pins.

INITIAL BONE MAPPING

This mapping is done by reproducing predefined 9 points for the femur and 7 points for the tibia **(Fig. 7.19)**. These points are specifically chosen by the operating surgeon on a preoperative 3D model of bone so that he can exactly reproduce these points. The error of recording these is reflected by RMSE. This

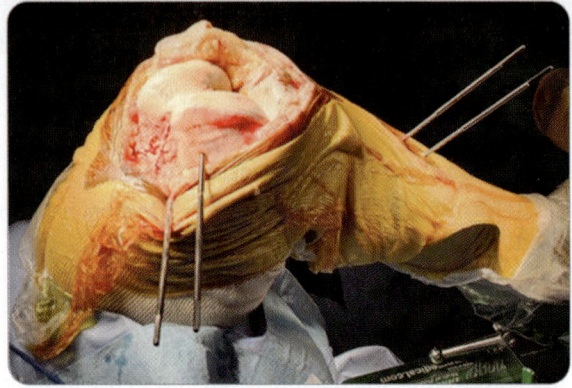

FIG. 7.18: Pin placement.

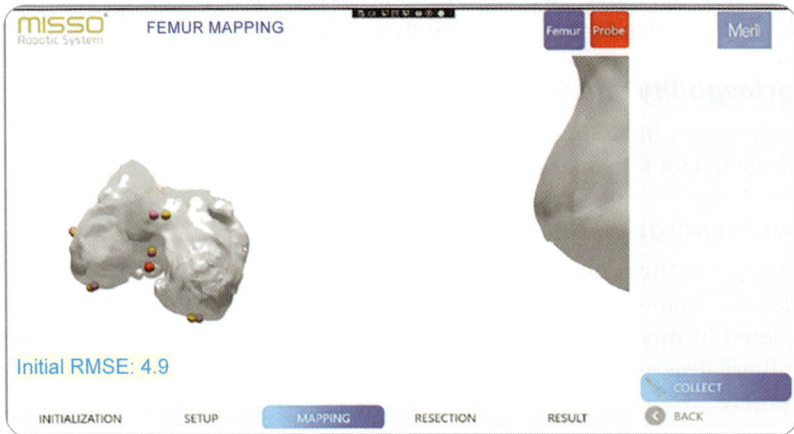

FIG. 7.19: Initial bone mapping.

value for initial bone mapping should be <10. If the initial RMSE is >10, repeat mapping should be done.

FINAL BONE MAPPING

After the initial bone mapping is done successfully, the final detailed mapping of bone must be done **(Fig. 7.20)**.

This requires 40 points in the femur and 40 points in the tibia. The final RMSE value should be below 1.

After final mapping verification of registration points are done. These verification points should be <1 mm of deviation.

GAP CHECK

After the final bone mapping of femur and tibia, gap checking is done **(Fig. 7.21)**. Extension gap check is done at near the extension. And the flexion gap check is done at 90° of flexion. Varus valgus stresses are applied to see maximum opening on the medial and lateral side.

Gap balancing values equal on both sides (9 mm) are achieved by adjusting the implants. In this step, mechanical alignment or restricted kinematic alignment, or kinematic alignment principles can be applied as per the surgeon's preference.

ROBOT PLACEMENT

After the gap balancing is achieved, the knee is fixed in flexion of 115°. As this is an active, autonomous cutting system, no bone movements are acceptable during bone cutting. To prevent such bone movement knee positioner (to hold the leg in a flexed position) and bone clamps or femoral/tibial pins (for bone holding) are used during the surgery. The robot is fixed near the operating table as per the instructions. The robot cart is on the ipsilateral side and the vision cart is placed on the opposite side **(Fig. 7.22)**.

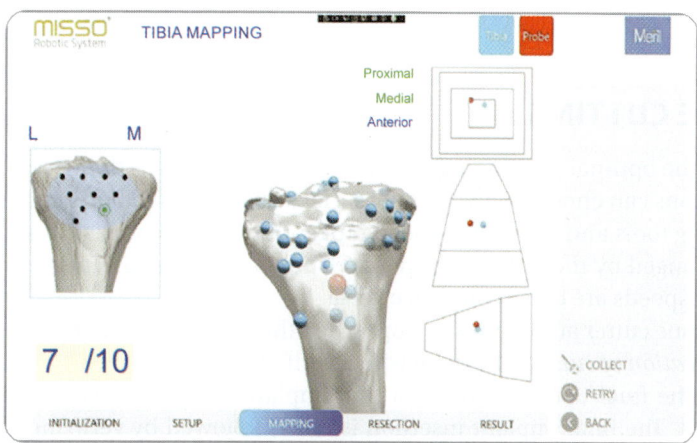

FIG. 7.20: Final bone mapping.

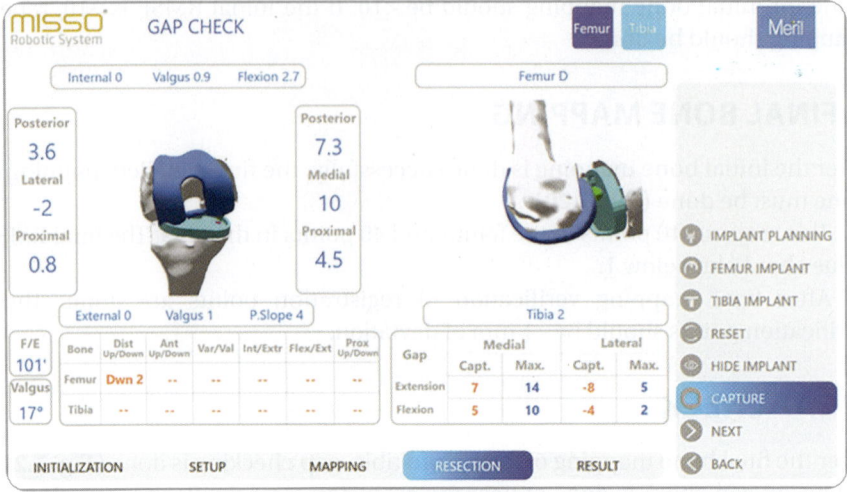

FIG. 7.21: Gap balancing.

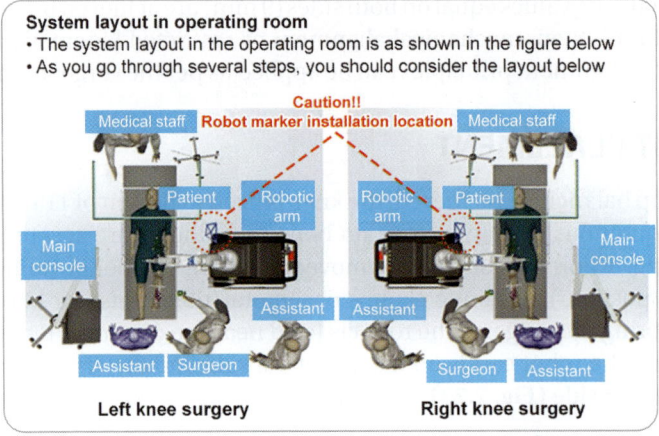

FIG. 7.22: Robot placement in the operation theater (OT) setup.

■ BONE CUTTING

- After the optimal positioning step by step, bone cutting is done **(Fig. 7.23)**.
- Surgeons can choose between only surface cutting or full bone cutting.
- Cutting tools and advancing speed ranges from 5 to 55 mm/s. This speed can be changed by the operator as per the surgeon's demands. In sclerotic bone, lower speeds are chosen and vice versa.
- The bone cutter automatically stops when the bone movement exceeds 2 mm. *Verification of cuts* can be done with a verification tool.

After the final cutting is done, a trial implant is inserted. Gap balancing is confirmed. The final implant insertion is done, followed by verifying gap check validation. Then markers and pins are removed.

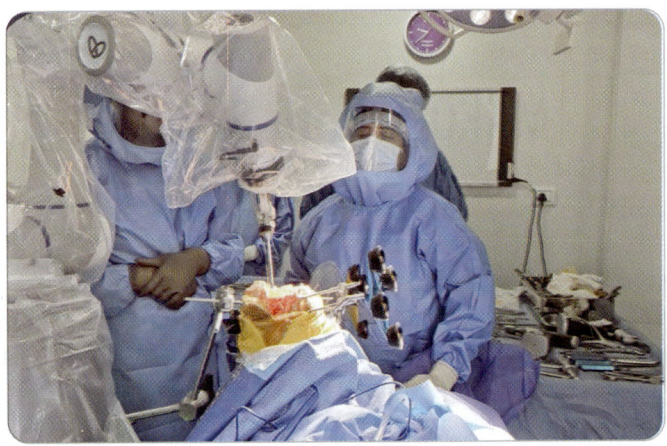

FIG. 7.23: Bone cutting process.

ADVANTAGES

- Being fully active with submillimeter precision, it has the upper hand over other robots other passive or semiactive robotic systems.
- Smaller human-like footprints are easy to work with, and also this robot can be accommodated in smaller OT setups.
- Due to the milling system, the prepared bone surface is even and without chip fractures, as sometimes seen in saw-based systems (may be seen in severe osteoporotic cases).
- Being developed in the local region, the cost burden is significantly lower.
- Cost per case is also significantly lower than comparable robotic systems.
- The development team is more accessible for innovative suggestions from surgeons. This may be reflected in making this system more promising.
- There are claims to incorporate trauma, spine, and arthroscopy in the same system.

DISADVANTAGES

- Being a fully active system, it takes more operational time than passive or semiactive systems.
- Being an image-based system needs a CT scan in every case. This exposes patients to radiation.

CONCLUSION

As MISSO is India's first indigenously developed robot has its own place in the robotic world. Moreover, it is a fully automated active system.

MAKO Robotic System

*Ajay Devda, Kathan Talsania, Sawankumar Pawar,
Sachin Yashwant Kale, Pramod Bhor*

INTRODUCTION

Haptics-using Robotic Arm Interactive Orthopedic System, like RIO from MAKO Stryker in Fort Lauderdale, Florida, received FDA approval in 2008. Recently published work on the results of robotically assisted total knee arthroplasty (TKA) has primarily focused on it. This system, when compared to other conventional techniques, results in reduced soft tissue trauma and postoperative pain, which reduces the number of hospital stays.

In 2017, Stryker, Mako Surgical Corp., USA, formally introduced the Mako Robotic-Arm Assisted System for main TKA, accelerating global adoption. Using a 3D model generated from preoperative CT scans, this image-dependent semi-active technique plans the size and orientation of the femoral and tibial components. During surgery, the presurgical plan is "mapped" to the patient's anatomy, enabling the operating surgeon to make any necessary adjustments. Due to haptic field limitations, the robotic arm can only remove bone that is within 0.5 mm of the original surgical plan.

It has been demonstrated that MAKO robotic arm-assisted operations can handle the technical difficulties that manual partial and/or multicompartmental knee treatments provide.

The end effector saw blade is autonomously positioned by the MAKO rigid arm in the proper resection plane and at a precise spot.

During and after the robotic arm-assisted treatment, data on component position, alignment, and soft tissue balance can be gathered, and these measurements may be used to predict the results of a total knee arthroplasty.

SYSTEM OVERVIEW: MAKO TKA SYSTEM

The Mako Navigation-assisted Robotic TKA system is used to consistently and reproducibly plan and execute a TKA.

CHAPTER 8: MAKO Robotic System

The Mako TKA system consists of the following tools and components **(Figs. 8.1 to 8.7)**:
- Robotic arm interactive orthopedic system (RIO)
- Optical tracking system with infrared camera stand and surgeon's console
- *Planning software workstation*: Guidance module
- Calibration and verification tools
- *Robotic arm attachment cutting system*: MICS (MAKO integrated cutting system) handpiece.

IMAGE OF ROBOTIC SYSTEM WITH LABELING

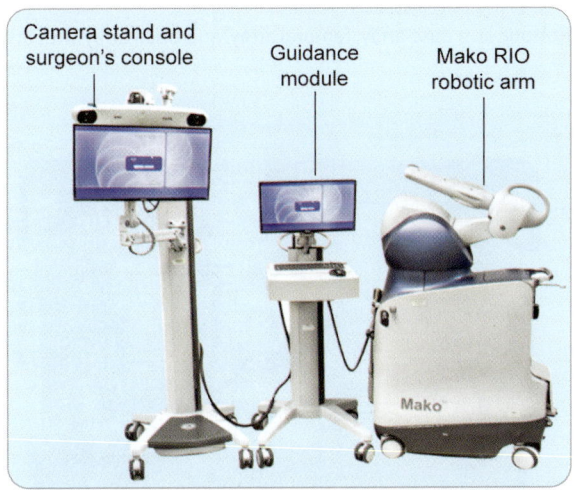

FIG. 8.1: MAKO robotic system including camera stand, guidance module, and RIO robotic arm.

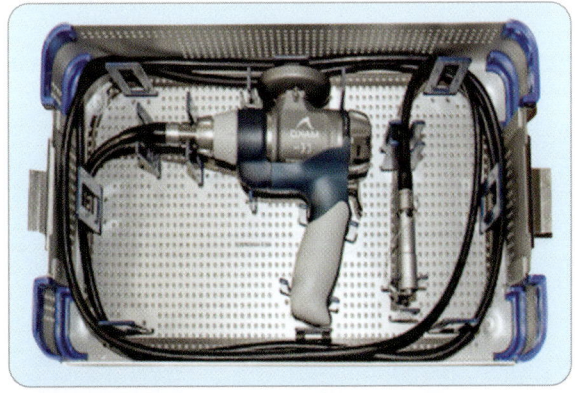

FIG. 8.2: MICS handpiece—cutting system that attaches to the robotic arm.

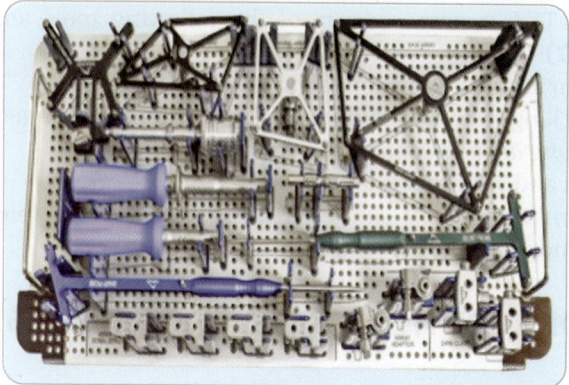

FIG. 8.3: Robotic arm base array, femoral array, and tibial array with attachments.

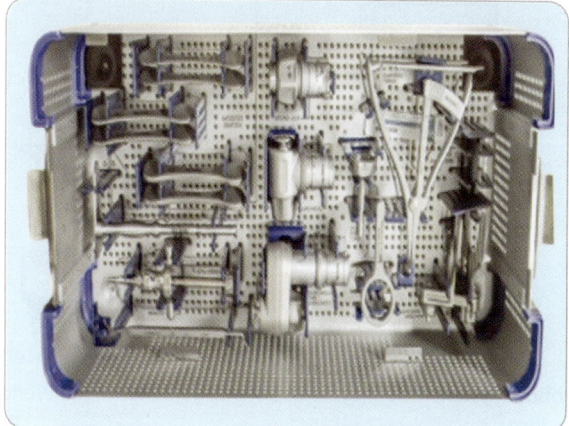

FIG. 8.4: Sagittal and right-angle saw attachments.

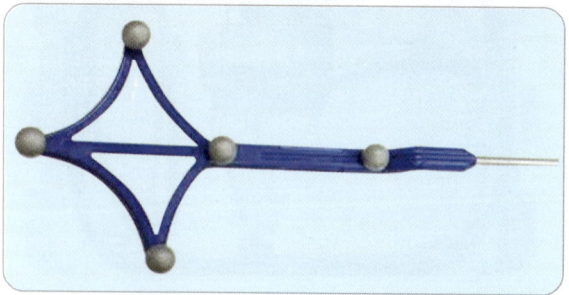

FIG. 8.5: Blunt and sharp probe with array adapters.

CHAPTER 8: MAKO Robotic System

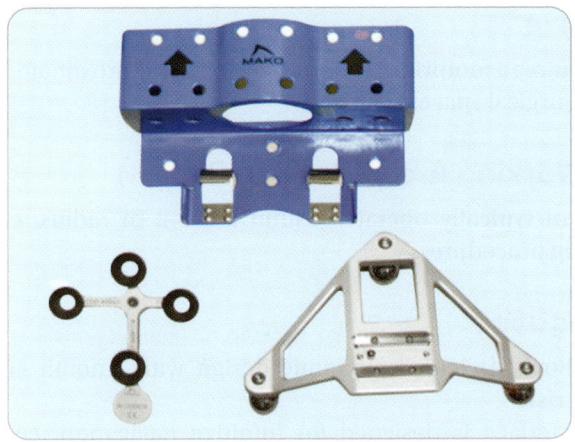

FIG. 8.6: Arm calibration attachments before draping.

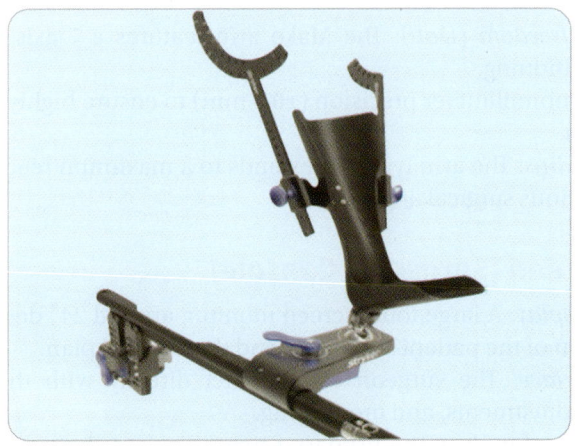

FIG. 8.7: Leg positioner with sled, boot, and rail clamp with retractors (antler).

■ STRYKER MAKO ROBOTIC SYSTEM SPECIFICATIONS

Size and Shape

Compact, upright design with a slim profile for easy maneuverability in operating rooms.
   Typically designed with a stable base and an extendable robotic arm.

Weight

The system weighs approximately 400–500 kg (varies slightly depending on model and configuration).

Footprint Size

The system requires a footprint of about 1.2 × 0.8 m (approximate size for optimal positioning in surgical spaces).

Minimum Working Area (Working Radius)

The robotic arm typically operates within a 1.5–2 m radius, ensuring ample flexibility during procedures.

Design Language

The system follows a clean, ergonomic design with smooth edges to reduce contamination risk.

The user interface is designed for intuitive navigation, combining touch screens and manual controls.

Robotic Arm Specifications

- *Degrees of freedom (DoF)*: The Mako arm features a 7-axis movement for precise positioning.
- *Accuracy*: Submillimeter precision (±0.5 mm) to ensure highly accurate bone preparation.
- *Working radius*: The arm typically extends to a maximum reach of about 1 m to cover various surgical angles.

Primary Screen (Surgeon's Console)

- *Size and display*: A large touchscreen monitor, around 24", designed for clear visualization of the patient's anatomy and the surgical plan.
- *Touch interface*: The surgeon can interact directly with the software for planning, adjustments, and monitoring.
- *Preoperative planning*: The primary screen displays the patient-specific 3D bone model based on the CT scan. The surgeon can interact with this screen to plan the surgery, adjust implant positioning, and assess alignment.
- *Intraoperative navigation*: It shows the real-time movement of the robotic arm during surgery, guiding bone resection and implant placement.
- *Surgical adjustments*: The surgeon can modify the plan or review key data, such as the alignment, range of motion, and stability of the joint, using the touchscreen interface.

Assistant Screen (Guidance Module)

- *Size and display*: This screen is generally smaller than the primary screen, around 19", but still offers clear visuals. This display is not a touchscreen.
- *System monitoring*: Displays critical system information, such as robotic arm calibration, status of bone registration, and real-time feedback on the accuracy of the procedure.

- *Robotic arm control*: Used by the surgical assistant or the Mako Product Specialist (MPS) to monitor robotic arm movements and assist with setup and adjustments, such as adjusting the surgical plan or responding to any technical alerts.
- *Maintenance and alerts*: The assistant screen is often used for monitoring alerts or system status, ensuring the robotic system is functioning optimally throughout the procedure.

Computed Tomography Scan

For the Mako TKA operation, every patient is required to have a preoperative CT scan. The Mako Knee CT Scanning Protocol (PN 200004) must be followed for this scan **(Table 8.1)**.

■ TIPS FOR COMPUTED TOMOGRAPHY SCAN

- Position the patient supine with their foot secured in an upright position (patella facing to the roof) using a rolled towel or blanket.
- Flex the knee slightly with a rolled towel or blanket.
- Wrap each Velcro strap around the rod (one at the hip and one at the ankle), completing a full revolution.

TABLE 8.1: CT scan requirements according to Mako CT scanning protocol (PN 200004).	
Scanner specifications	- *Type*: Multidetector CT (MDCT) scanner (64-slice or higher) - *Slice thickness*: 0.625 mm (ideal for precise bone mapping), 0.5–1 mm is acceptable - *Reconstruction interval*: 0.3–0.5 mm overlap for enhanced detail
Patient positioning	- *Supine position* with the surgical limb in neutral alignment - Use a *foot holder or knee bolster* to maintain alignment - Ensure the hip and knee joints are in a natural, extended position
Imaging parameters	- *KV (Kilovoltage)*: 120–140 kV - *mAs (Milliampere-seconds)*: Adjust per patient size (typically 150–300 mAs) - *Bone kernel*: High-resolution bone algorithm (e.g., B70 or B75) - *Window setting*: Bone window (e.g., 2,000 HU width, 500 HU level)
Data format	- Export in *DICOM format* (mandatory for Mako software integration), ensuring *continuous, nongapped slices* without missing data - No metal artifacts—ensure metal implants are accounted for during scanning
Knee region	Scan minimum of 10 cm above and below the distal femoral condyles, including the margin above the patellofemoral joint and margin below the tibial tuberosity, with the center being around the joint line
Scanning time-period	Anytime before surgery up to 8 weeks

- Place the motion rod from just above the hip-center to below the ankle-center.
- Adjust femoral and tibial additional straps to secure the rod.
- Ensure the rod is visible in both the anterior/posterior and medial/lateral fields of view. The Velcro straps should be snug but not too tight.

STRYKER MAKO OPTICAL TRACKING SYSTEM DETAILS

- *Camera specifications*:
  - *Type*: Infrared camera with high-precision tracking capabilities
  - *Manufacturer*: Typically sourced from leading medical imaging tech providers (e.g., Northern Digital Inc. or similar)
  - *Vision angle*: Wide-angle lens, offering a field of view of approximately 60–90° for optimal room coverage
- *Optical trackers*:
  - *Type*: Passive spherical markers (reflective) for enhanced precision and reduced interference.
  - *Design*: Spherical markers for improved visibility from multiple angles.
  - *Lifespan*: Durable with extended usability; typically replaced when worn or damaged.
- *Plane formation (arrays/markers)*:
  - *Formation*: Multiplane array system designed to track instrument position relative to the surgical site.
  - *Number of planes*: Typically, two to three planes to ensure full 3D spatial awareness.
- *Margin of error*: Achieves submillimeter precision, typically around ± 0.5 mm, ensuring highly accurate bone preparation and implant positioning.
- *Interactive device (monitor specifications)*:
  - *Type*: High-definition medical-grade touchscreen monitor
  - *Size*: Typically, 21–27" for clear visualization
  - *Resolution*: Full HD or 4K UHD for precise surgical mapping
  - *Interface*: Intuitive UI with real-time visual guidance, anatomical overlays, and adjustable view angles.

STRYKER MAKO CUTTING SYSTEM DETAILS

Type

The Mako cutting system for TKA utilizes an oscillating saw blade system with two different attachments to the MICS handpiece for precise bone resection with minimal soft tissue disruption. The ideal attachment is a straight saw attachment, and another is a sagittal saw attachment.

The straight saw attachment is used for anterior femur cut, anterior chamfer cut, posterior femoral cuts, and tibial cut, while the sagittal saw attachment is used for distal femur cut and posterior chamfer cut.

Cutter Blade Specifications (Figs. 8.8 and 8.9)

- *Size*: It comes in two sizes, narrow blade cutting edge is 9 mm (Mako saw blade 116171) and the ideal blade comes with cutting edge of 18 mm (Mako saw blade 116170) which can cover up to 25 mm area while oscillating for cutting and the thickness of both the blade is 2 mm.
- *Material*: Made from titanium for durability and precision.
- *Design*: The blade edge is sharp and precise with cutting edges as shown in **Figures 8.8 and 8.9**.

Speed and Control

Operating at a speed of 1,500–3,000 oscillations/min, ensuring precise bone sculpting with minimal heat generation.

Speed is dynamically controlled based on the surgeon's inputs and the system's safety protocols to prevent over-resection.

Safety Features

The system is programmed with haptic boundaries, preventing the saw from cutting beyond the predefined surgical plan.

Real-time visual and auditory feedback alerts the surgeon if deviation occurs.

PLANNING METHODOLOGY OF MAKO TKA SOFTWARE APPLICATION (STEP-BY-STEP PROCESS) (FIG. 8.10)

Step 1: The login page

Enter the "Username" and "Password" and select the "Login" button. The available user types include Clinical User (surgeon), Administrator (MAKO product specialist), and service agent.

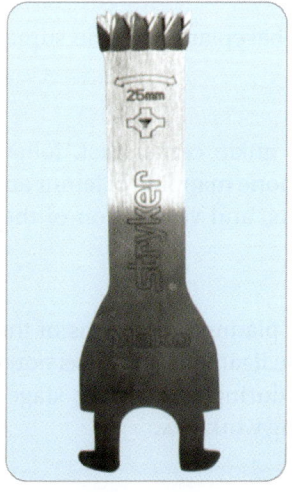

FIG. 8.8: Mako saw blade 116170 (normal).

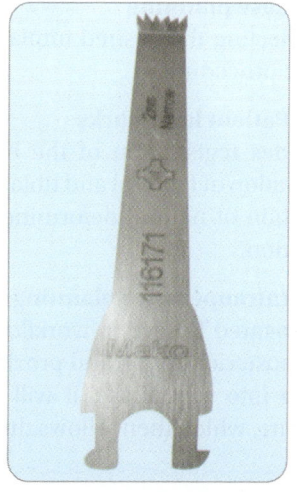

FIG. 8.9: Mako saw blade 116171 (narrow).

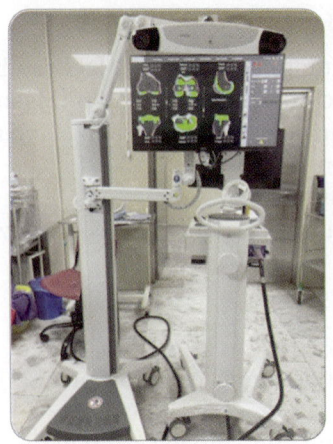 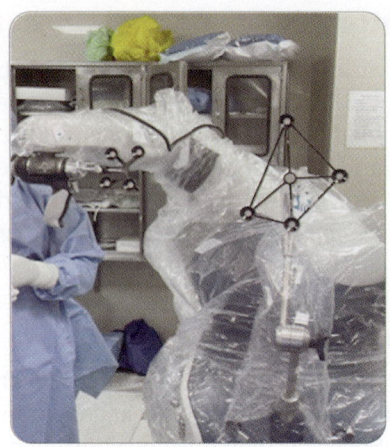

FIG. 8.10: MAKO navigation system.   **FIG. 8.11:** MAKO robotic arm.

Step 2: Surgery selection
The starting page after login will display the options of the surgical plans between PKA, THA, and TKA. Select TKA as a surgical plan.

Step 3: Plan management
The next step is plan management, where multiple options will be available to import the surgical plan of TKA by USB method to import/remove/delete/archive/unarchive. Import the plan from the USB drive with the surgical plan attached to the monitor **(Fig. 8.11)**.

Step 4: Import DICOM
The next step is to import the CT scan images of the patient and review the DICOM images. Select the "check for motion" tab, and the software checks the patient scan for any irregularities caused by patient motion during the scan.

Step 5: Case planning
After selecting the desired implant system and baseplate type, the surgeon can start the procedure.

Step 6: Patient landmarks
It includes registration of the hip center and ankle center first, followed by implantation of femoral and tibial checkpoints, bone mapping of femur and tibia, registration of natural deformities of knee joints, and verification of the entire registration.

Step 7: Intraoperative planning
The Measured Resection workflow involves the planned resections of the distal femur, posterior femur, and proximal tibia. While ligament tension is not directly factored into this phase, it will be evaluated during the trialing stage of the procedure, which then follows the joint balancing workflow.

Step 8: Intraoperative planning
It includes the implant planning page, which provides the surgeon one last opportunity to modify the plan based on the limb alignment assessment performed in the "Joint Balancing" page.

Step 9: Bone preparation
The RIO system is moved to the desired position as per the software allowance near the table, and bone preparations can be initiated after rechecking of check-points on the bone and a checkpoint on the attached blade with the MICS handpiece.

Step 10: Trial implantation and final results
After successful bone preparation by the RIO robotic arm, the surgeon can put the trial implants in and check for the gap balancing in flexion and extension. The alignment, stability, and range of motion are carefully evaluated. It can also show the complete range of motion and achievable full flexion of the knee joint. Throughout the procedure, the leg is stabilized with a leg holding device **(Fig. 8.12)**.

STRYKER MAKO TKA SURGICAL STEPS

Insertion of a Bone Pin (Tibia Only)
- Using a scalpel, make a single incision through the skin and fascia between 1 and 1.5 cm medial to the tibial crest and at least 10 cm (about four fingerbreadths) inferior to the tibial tubercle **(Fig. 8.13)**.
- One of the two techniques listed below can be used to finish the second incision: Make the second stab incision around 15 mm away from the first one, or, alternatively, insert the Array Stabilizer's most proximal sleeve through the first incision and make an incision where the distal sleeve sits on the skin.
- Insert the Array Stabilizer completely through both incisions, making sure the barrels are on the surface of the bone.

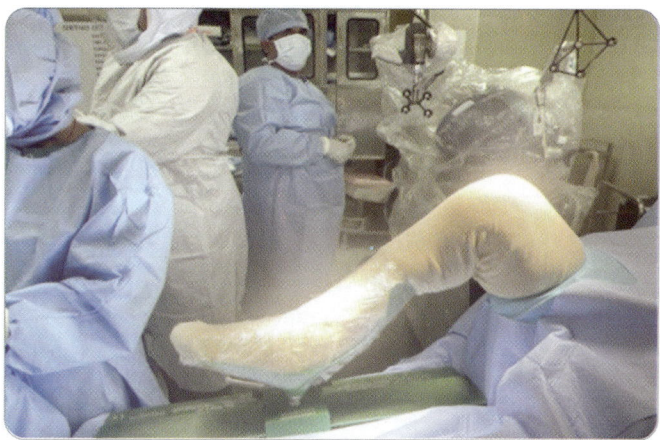

FIG. 8.12: Leg positioner kit on the table.

- Use one of the bone pins to pierce the second cortex after passing through the first cortex at approximately a 45° angle from the sagittal midline.
- Insert the second bone pin through the first cortex and pierce the second cortex while holding the Array Stabilizer in place.

INSERTION OF BONE PINS (ONLY FEMUR)

- To lengthen the quadriceps muscles, bend the knee beyond 90°.
- With a scalpel and at least 9–10 cm (four fingerbreadths) above the superior edge of the patella, create a single incision through the skin and fascia.
- *One of the two techniques listed below can be used to complete the second incision*: Make the second stab incision about 15 mm away from the first one, or, alternatively, insert the array stabilizer's distalmost sleeve through the first incision and make an incision where the proximal sleeve sits on the skin **(Fig. 8.14)**.
- Insert the femoral pins through the array stabilizer completely through both incisions, making sure the barrels are on the surface of the bone at an ideal angle of 30° medial from midline sagittal.
- Insert the second bone pin through the first cortex and pierce the second cortex while holding the array stabilizer in place.

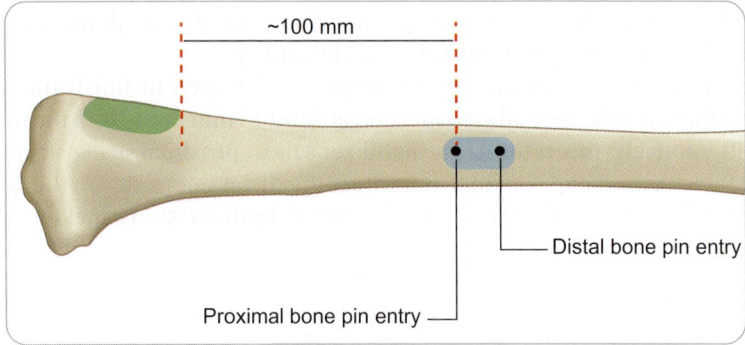

FIG. 8.13: Position of tibia pin insertion.

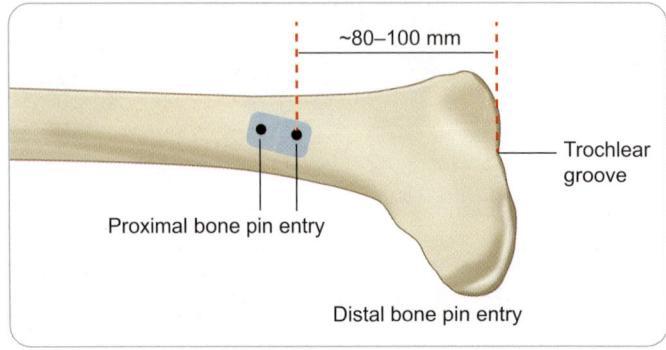

FIG. 8.14: Position of femoral pin insertion.

ARRAY ASSEMBLY (FEMUR AND TIBIA)

- Loosely assemble the 2-pin clamp and array adaptor.
- After passing the clamp over the bone pins, the top of the array stabilizer is pressed against the clamp. Position the assembly so that the screw on the clamp faces away from the camera and the screw on the Array Adaptor faces away from the incision.
- Join the Array Adaptor to the knee femoral array.
- Set the array's position as desired.
- Tighten the screws in the following order, using the square driver: A screw for an array, a screw for an array adaptor, and a clamp screw.

INCISION/ARTHROTOMY

Done according to the surgeon's preference.

The Leg Positioner and Self-Retraction System are both optional. The stereotactic boundary used to restrict the saw blade is generated based on the implant size, shape, and plan.

The Robotic Arm does not have the ability to track a patient's soft tissues. It is recommended to use standard retraction techniques during robotic arm-assisted cutting.

REGISTRATION AND VERIFICATION OF BONES

It starts with patient landmarks registration, including hip center, and ankle center (medial and lateral malleolus) **(Fig. 8.15)**.

For medial malleolus: Collect the point by palpating the anterior and posterior surfaces of the medial malleolus and place the blunt probe (Green) tip in the center and "Capture".

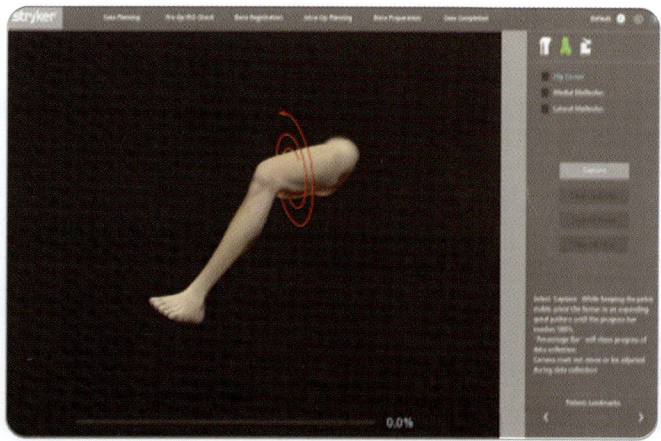

FIG. 8.15: Hip center verification screen.

For lateral malleolus: Collect the point by palpating the anterior and posterior surfaces of the lateral malleolus and place the blunt probe (Green) tip in the center and "Capture".

Tip: While collecting the malleolus landmarks, do not reposition the leg and ankle.

The registration patterns for the femur and tibia both have 40 points (10 groups of four points each). Setting the anteroposterior (AP), mediolateral (ML), proximal/distal directions, and axial rotation (internal/external) alignment of each bone depends heavily on the points. Registration of bone mapping is done with the pointed probe (blue) by putting the pointed end on the bone at almost the same position shown in the Mako display system. When a CT scan is used to create the patient-specific model and only the bone structure is segmented, as a result, points for bone registration must be gathered on the bone.

Tip: Use the Sharp Probe to pierce the cartilage and stop on the bone surface when points are collected in areas that are coated in cartilage.

If the points are marked on the osteophytes, then do not pierce the osteophyte to collect the point.

Femur checkpoint **(Fig. 8.16A)**: Ensure that the femur checkpoint is placed in hard bone and located approximately 10 mm away from the nearest femur cut. Collect and verify the checkpoint.

Tibia checkpoint **(Fig. 8.16B)**: Ensure that the tibia checkpoint is placed in hard bone and located approximately 10 mm away from the tibia cut. Collect and verify the checkpoint.

For verifications of the bone mapping, touch the tip of the blue probe to the point on the bone corresponding to one of the larger blue spheres displayed on screen **(Figs. 8.17 and 18)**. Located to the right of the model are guides displaying the probe.

Distance to bone in mm and a 2D CT slice of the bone contour. Press "Verify". The software will display an accuracy value (depending on the set surgeon's preference) of the measured distance between the probe tip and the registered bone model. If the accuracy value for that point is within the acceptable limit, a sound will play, and the blue point will turn white, signifying that the bone

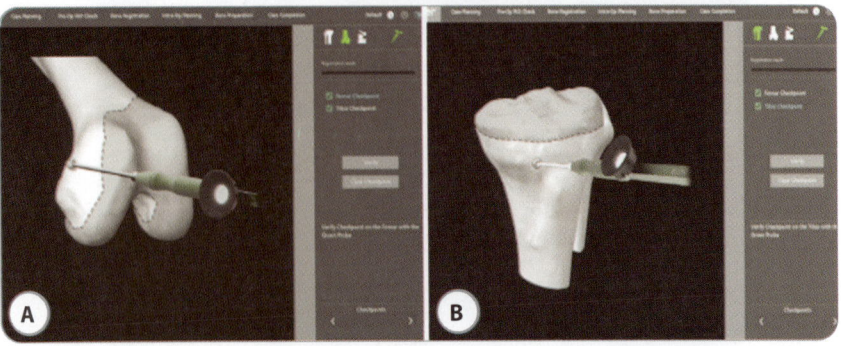

FIGS. 8.16A AND B: Femoral and tibial checkpoints position and verification screen.

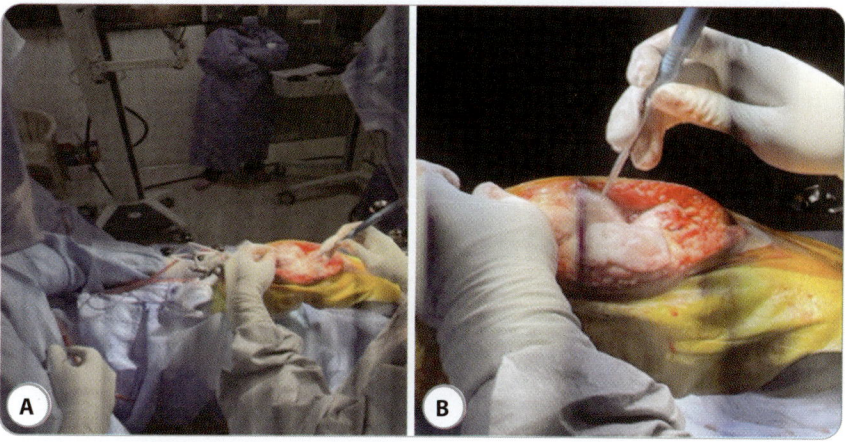

FIGS. 8.17A AND B: Intraoperative bone surface marking.

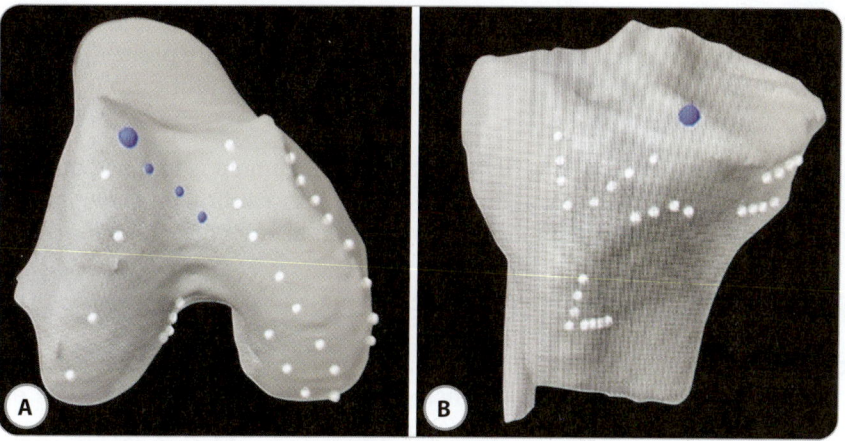

FIGS. 8.18A AND B: Intraoperative bone surface marking on navigation screen.

registration at the point is accurate. If the blue point turns red, the accuracy value was found to be above the acceptable limit.

Repeat for all six verification points for the final accuracy value. This final verification step is crucial and necessary. It decreases the root mean square errors.

JOINT BALANCING AND IMPLANT PLANNING

The "Joint Balancing" provides real-time limb alignment to assess the knee joint. Clinical and mechanical deformities such as flexion, recurvatum, fixed varus/valgus deformity, and limited flexion may require intra-operative changes for the implant planning **(Fig. 8.19)**.

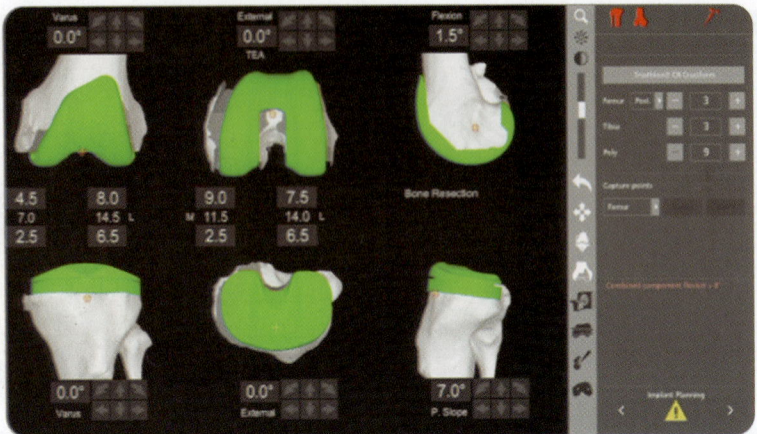

FIG. 8.19: Preoperative implant planning and positioning according to computed tomography (CT) scan.

Tip: An alternate method to verify tibia axial rotation is to place the thumb and index finger on either side of the tibial tubercle, place the sharp probe tip between the two fingers, and visually confirm onscreen that the probe tip is centrally located on the tibial tubercle.

Tip: An alternate method to verify tibia coronal alignment is to place the Sharp Probe on the medial and lateral malleoli and visually confirm on-screen that the tip is the same distance from the medial malleolus as from the lateral malleolus.

BALANCING PRIOR TO RESECTION

Prior to performing any bone resections, the projected gaps are balanced using a method called "Preresection balancing **(Fig. 8.20)**". Several techniques exist for preresection joint tensioning, such as Paddles to apply tension to one or both compartments, osteotomes to apply tension to one or both compartments with knee valgus or varus movement to exert strain on a single compartment **(Figs. 8.21 and 8.22)**.

BONY PREPARATION

For the preferred cutting workflow, choose the desired bone cut. On the "Surgeon preferences" page, each surgeon can specify how the bone cuts should be made. For the "Measured Resection" workflow to be as efficient as possible, with the least amount of checkpoints and saw attachment modifications, the following cutting order is advised.

By a straight saw attachment to the MICS handpiece:
- *First*: Femur anterior cut
- *Second*: Femur anterior chamfer cut
- *Third*: Femur posterior cuts
- *Fourth*: Proximal tibial cut

CHAPTER 8: MAKO Robotic System

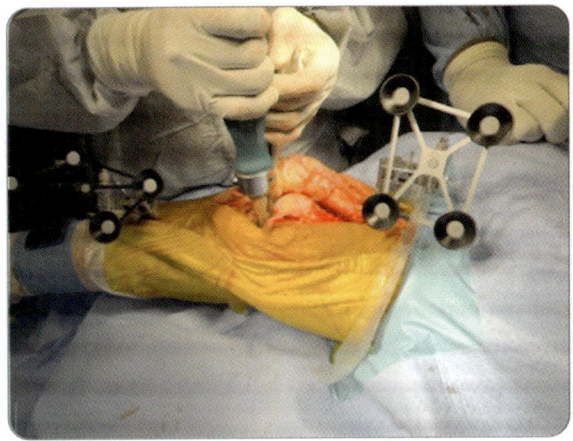

FIG. 8.20: Intraoperative sensors on femur and tibia with bone marking sensor where the surgeon is holding spacers for preresection gap balancing.

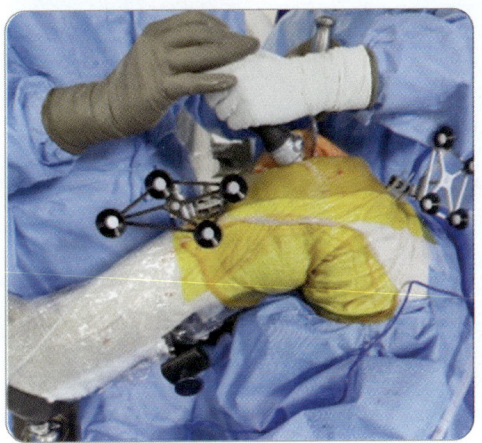

FIG. 8.21: Ligamental tensioning with spacers.

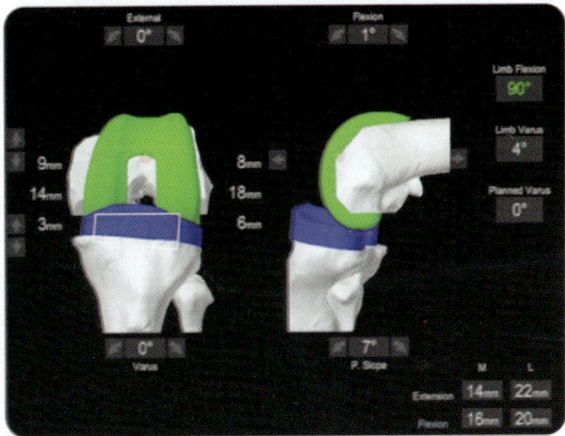

FIG. 8.22: Ligamental tensioning in display system.

By a sagittal saw attachment to the MICS handpiece:
- *Fifth*: Femur distal cut
- *Sixth*: Femur posterior chamfer cut

Use the on-screen instructions to complete the resection and remove all of the green-appearing bone. "Extended boundary" should be used if all the bone that needs to be removed cannot be reached.

POSTRESECTION BALANCING

Postbony resection gap balancing in extension and flexion will be measured after putting a trial implant **(Figs. 8.23 and 8.24)**.

FINAL IMPLANTATION

Refer **Figures 8.25A to C**.

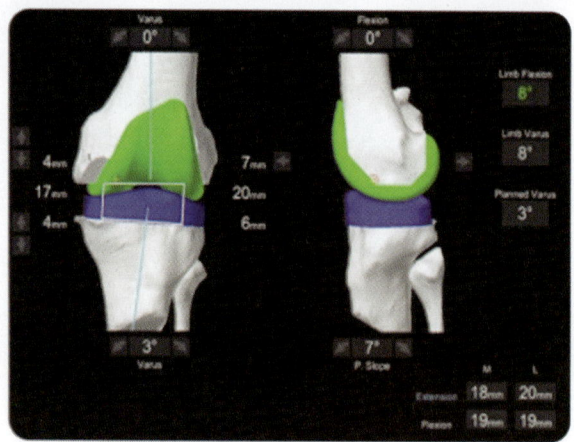

FIG. 8.23: Post-trial implant ligamental balancing in extension.

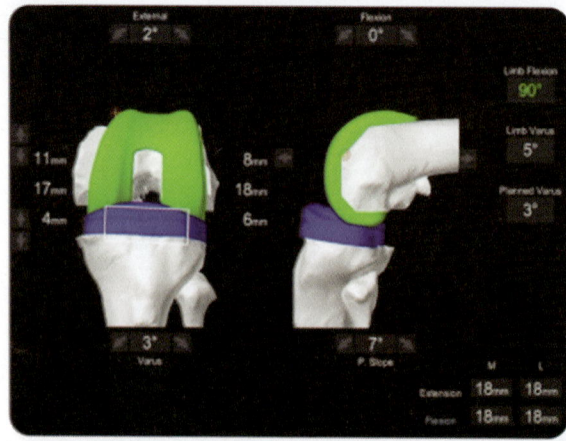

FIG. 8.24: Post-trial implant ligamental balancing in flexion.

CHAPTER 8: MAKO Robotic System 83

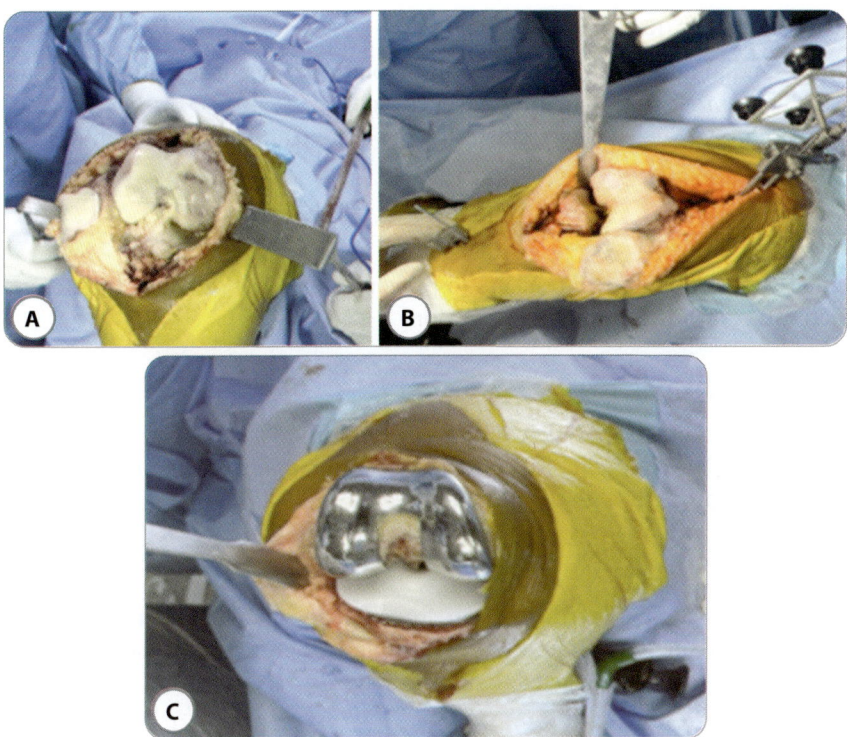

FIGS. 8.25A TO C: Arthritic knee preimplantation.

MAKO TIPS AND TRICKS: THE PRACTICAL GUIDE

Robot Placement in Operating Theater

Position the Mako system on the opposite side of the surgical team to maintain a clear workspace.

The robotic arm should be aligned to maximize its working radius without restricting the surgeon's movement.

Ensure the optical tracking camera is placed at an elevated angle for optimal marker visibility.

If desired, the robot can be moved away from the surgical table until the bone preparation step.

Pin Placement

Always place pins perpendicular to the bone. Ensure they are secure and away from the planned cutting zone to maintain tracking accuracy.

While tightening the array clamps, make sure to hold them with another hand to stabilize them and avoid any pin breakage.

Patient Landmark Registration

Reduce medial and lateral motion of the hip joint by securing the pelvis during the hip center registration to improve accuracy.

Do not move the leg while registering the medial and lateral malleolus (ankle center).

Optical Tracker Hygiene

Regularly clean the optical trackers to prevent bony dust or blood interference, which can compromise tracking precision.

Bone Mapping

Carefully identify and mark key anatomical landmarks such as the medial and lateral epicondyles and femoral condyles. Accurate mapping ensures the robotic system aligns properly with the preoperative CT model.

Gap Balancing

Maintain consistent joint distraction force during gap balancing to achieve uniform soft tissue tension and optimal implant alignment. Instead of paddles, the osteotomes can also be used to do distraction.

Leg Positioning

For knee replacements, maintain 90° flexion during the mapping and cutting phases. The position of the leg holder is also very important, and make sure to tighten and recheck all the clamps on the leg positioner. Place the leg positioner in such a way that performing flexion and extension at the knee joint becomes easy.

Using a side support can interfere with the Mako robot's position.

Cutting

Use slow, controlled hand movements during cutting to prevent chatter marks and ensure a smooth bone surface. Follow the designated cutting path within the haptic boundaries for optimal precision.

Trial Reduction

Always perform a trial reduction post-cutting to confirm proper implant alignment, stability, and range of motion before final implantation.

Robot Over-reliance

While the Mako system enhances precision, manual oversight is crucial. Always verify critical steps such as pin stability, bone mapping accuracy, and implant positioning.

Final Thought

Combining precise robotic control with sound surgical judgment ensures optimal patient outcomes and minimizes intraoperative errors.

Robotic Mako knee replacement surgery represents a significant advancement in orthopedic care, combining precision, accuracy, and personalized planning to achieve optimal outcomes. By integrating detailed CT-based mapping with robotic guidance, the Mako system empowers surgeons to deliver consistent and reproducible results. This technology not only enhances implant positioning and alignment but also contributes to improved joint function and patient satisfaction.

As robotic-assisted surgery continues to evolve, Mako stands at the forefront, offering a refined approach that prioritizes both surgical precision and patient well-being.

CONCLUSION

With compelling evidence of less pain and improved long-term results, Mako TKR offers substantial advantages over manual TKR in terms of accuracy, recovery time, and patient satisfaction. However, some significant disadvantages include its higher cost, learning curve, and reliance on particular implants and training. To determine suitability and go over possible risks, like infection or blood clots, which are still comparable to manual methods, patients thinking about Mako TKR should speak with a qualified orthopedic surgeon.

CHAPTER 9

VELYS Robotic System

Santosh Shetty, Pramod Bhor, Sachin Yashwant Kale, Sawankumar Pawar, Syed Mussadique Ali, Gaurav Patel, Raj M Sawant

INTRODUCTION

The VELYS™ Robotic-Assisted Solution (VRAS) is designed to enhance surgical precision by integrating CT-free technology to optimize implant placement. This system equips surgeons with the information needed to preserve the soft tissue envelope, predict joint stability, and work toward returning knee function. It is manufactured by Johnson and Johnson MedTech—DePuy Orthopedics.

VELYS™ Robotic-Assisted Solutions is the fourth generation of robotic-assisted devices. It endorses a patient-specific alignment philosophy in total knee replacement (TKR) for improved precision and accuracy personalized for each patient's specific anatomy. Fully controlled by the surgeon during surgery, the robot helps to provide surgical insights for real-time decision making with free movement and precise access to the affected knee joint.

VELYS™ Robotic-Assisted Solutions has won the REDDOT 2021 Award **(Fig. 9.1)** for its compact system design that is strikingly emphasized by its slim profiles and narrow radii.

"In search of good design"—the Red Dot Design Award is one of the world's largest design competitions. The Red Dot Label has become established internationally as one of the most sought-after marks of quality for good design.

The VELYS™ Robotic System offers a simple yet versatile workflow that complements the surgeon's current workflow, is easily adaptable, and is designed in a manner where a surgeon can plan, execute, and perform the surgery with great ease. It simplifies knee replacement surgery by providing valuable insights, versatile execution, and verified performance designed to deliver efficiency for surgeons and optimize patient outcomes. This proprietary technology maintains the saw cut plane to help execute precise, reproducible surgeon-controlled cuts.

The VELYS™ Robotic-Assisted Solution works exclusively with the ATTUNE™ Knee System, which has been used by over 1 million patients worldwide and is designed to deliver a greater range of motion (ROM) and faster recovery, and greater functional outcomes.

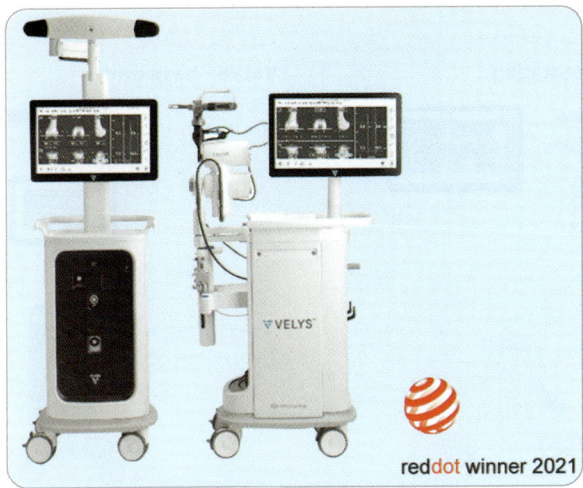

FIG. 9.1: VELYS™ Robotic System (REDDOT Award Winner 2021).

KEY FEATURES OF THE VELYS™ ROBOTIC-ASSISTED SOLUTIONS

- *Computed tomography (CT)-free technology*: The VRAS utilizes CT-free technology to help surgeons perform replacement procedures and place implants with precision and accuracy. The elimination of the CT scan results in shorter operative time and a higher degree of patient safety, as the patients are not exposed to radiation.
- *Real-time data system*: The VELYS™ robot presents real-time intraoperative images using a high-speed camera and motion technology, providing insights for real-time decision making. It enables the surgeon to precisely remove arthritic cartilage and ensure balanced tension in the knee throughout the ROM, allowing accurate positioning of the knee implant.
- *Adaptive planning*: The VRAS helps the surgeon to plan and personalize alignment based on the patient's specific anatomy, allowing an effective knee replacement best suited for each patient.

ROBOT DIMENSIONS AND WEIGHT

Refer **Table 9.1**.

SHAPE AND ERGONOMIC DESIGN

Space in the operating room (OR) is a valuable commodity, one that should not be compromised. Because certain robotic-assisted system equipment can take up much-needed space in the OR and limit the space in the room to move for the OR staff, it is advantageous to incorporate a system that minimizes space requirements to maximize surgical efficiencies.

CHAPTER 9: VELYS Robotic System

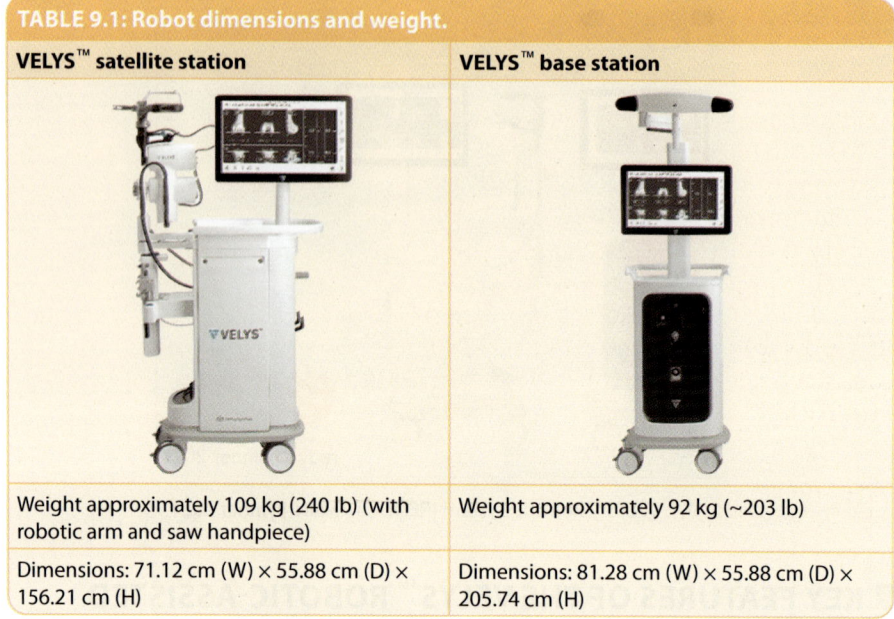

TABLE 9.1: Robot dimensions and weight.

VELYS™ satellite station	VELYS™ base station
Weight approximately 109 kg (240 lb) (with robotic arm and saw handpiece)	Weight approximately 92 kg (~203 lb)
Dimensions: 71.12 cm (W) × 55.88 cm (D) × 156.21 cm (H)	Dimensions: 81.28 cm (W) × 55.88 cm (D) × 205.74 cm (H)

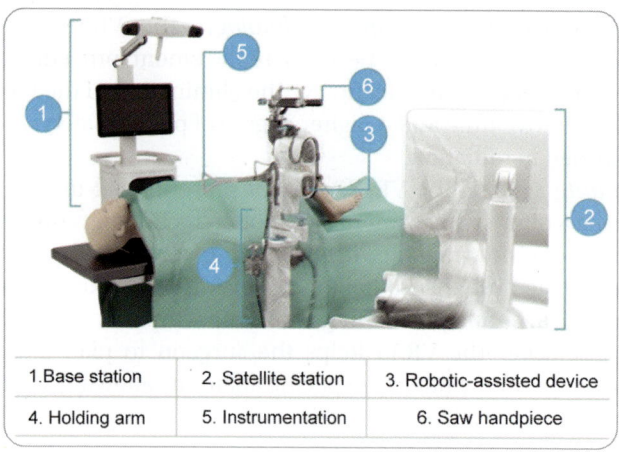

1. Base station	2. Satellite station	3. Robotic-assisted device
4. Holding arm	5. Instrumentation	6. Saw handpiece

FIG. 9.2: Main components of the VELYS™ Robotic System.

VELYS™ robotic system **(Fig 9.2)** is undoubtedly the most compact design available, and the robotic operation does not depend on the availability of a company-trained robotic specialist, enabling optimum use of OT space.

Moreover, the robotic arm that gets attached to the bedrail has the thinnest profile; it does not interfere in a way of surgery when the surgeon needs to make an incision or take out osteophytes or access the joint space. The compactness of the robotic arm in the sterile field improves OR flow and surgical access.

The robotic saw, mounted on a robotic arm, has a surgeon trolled trigger that gets activated only in the surgical plane. It is not too bulky and mimics the function as of the manual saw, making its adaptation easy in practice.

BASE STATION SPECIFICATIONS (FIG. 9.3)

VELYS™ Camera

VELYS™ has a high-speed camera **(Fig. 9.4)** that refreshes itself at the speed of 250 Hertz (Hz) per second. This allows the camera and the software to track leg movement during the surgery and adjust the cutting plane accordingly.

The camera has an infrared tracking system. It determines the location of each array in three-dimensional space.

VELYS™ works on adaptive tracking technology that uses high-speed camera, triple-drive motion technology, and PURESIGHT™ Hydrophobic Optical Reflectors work together to adjust and control the resection plane for accurate, consistent execution of to plan. The camera works on infrared light reflected from PURESIGHT Hydrophobic Optical Markers/Reflectors **(Fig. 9.5)**.

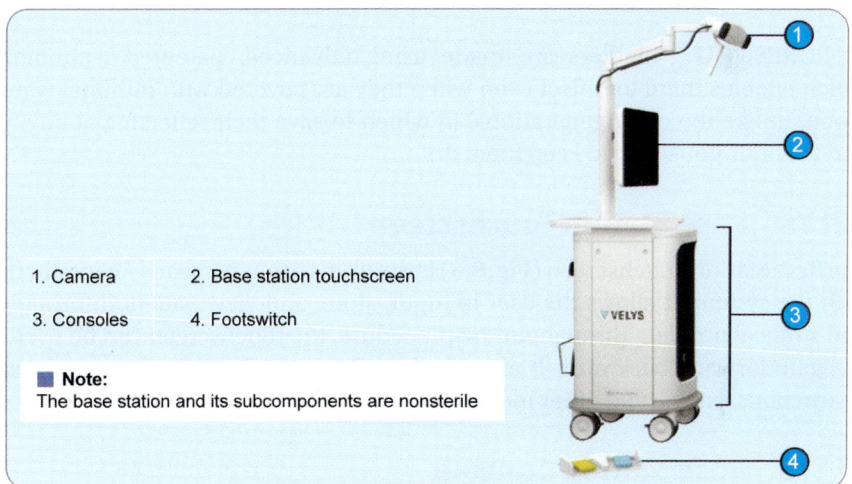

1. Camera
2. Base station touchscreen
3. Consoles
4. Footswitch

Note:
The base station and its subcomponents are nonsterile

FIG. 9.3: The Base Station and its components.

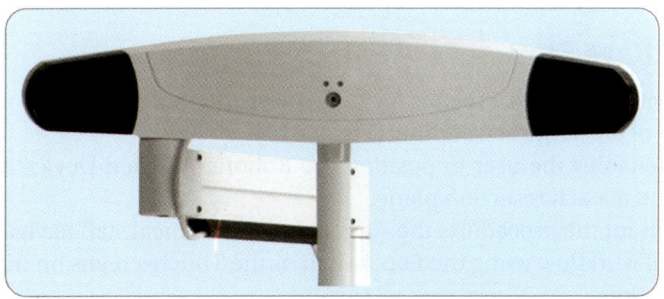

FIG. 9.4: VELYS™ Camera.

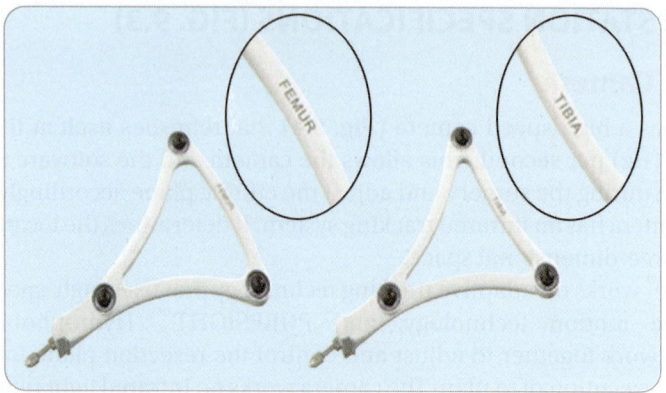

FIG. 9.5: PURESIGHT hydrophobic optical markers of Femur and Tibia. Distance needed to maintain between the camera from the reflector markers is minimum 6 ft.

PURESIGHT™ markers are made using advanced, patented technology, which enables them to reflect even when they are covered with minimal water/blood, unlike the older generations, in which to save their reflecting ability, we had to continuously try to keep them dry.

VELYS™ Base Station Touchscreen

The Base Station Touchscreen **(Fig. 9.6)** is the user's primary means for interacting with the system. It allows the user to input, store, and view patient information and surgical profiles. Throughout the procedure, the touchscreen can be used to navigate forward/backward. It also displays information to the user, including instructions, errors, and other messages.

VELYS™ Base Station Console

The Base Station contains integrated consoles **(Fig. 9.7)**. These consoles drive the Robotic-Assisted Device, Saw, Camera, Touchscreen, and Footswitch and execute the software.

VELYS™ Base Station Footswitch

The footswitch provides a means for hands-free interaction with the system and navigation of the surgical workflow **(Fig. 9.8)**.

It also enables the user to position the Robotic-Assisted Device at its home position and at each resection plane.

Throughout the procedure, the surgeon and/or clinical staff navigate through the surgical workflow using the Footswitch or the Touchscreens on the Base and Satellite Stations.

CHAPTER 9: VELYS Robotic System

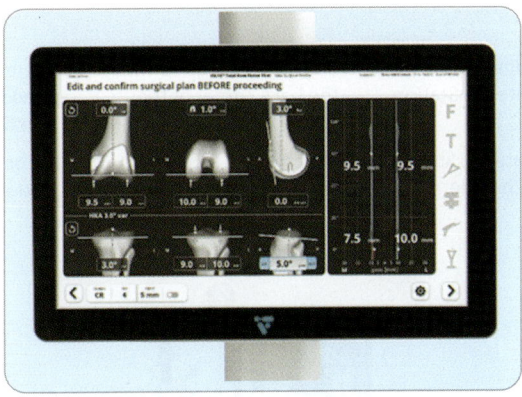

FIG. 9.6: Base Station Touchscreen.

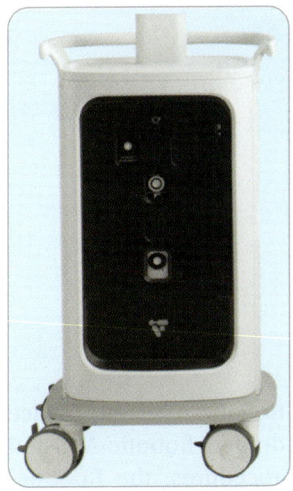

FIG. 9.7: VELYS™ Base Station Console.

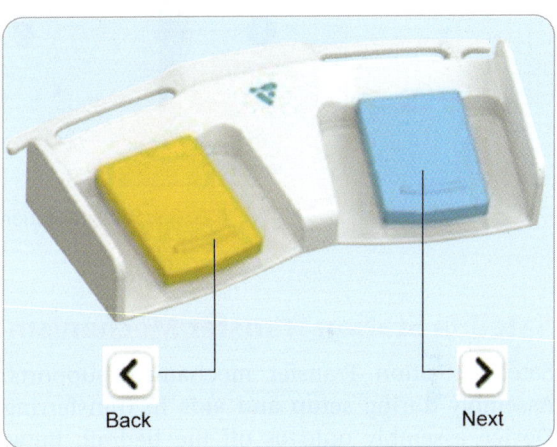

FIG. 9.8: VELYS™ Base Station Footswitch.

SATELLITE STATION SPECIFICATIONS (TABLE 9.2)

The Satellite Station **(Fig. 9.9)** (including the touchscreen) is covered by a sterile drape for the entire procedure, allowing the surgeon to interact with the user interface directly, if desired.

Satellite Station Touchscreen

The Satellite Station Touchscreen mirrors the Base Station Touchscreen display. No difference (refer to the base screen touchscreen in **Figure 9.6**).

TABLE 9.2: Explaining the details of Satellite Station as discussed in Figure 9.9.

A. Front of the Satellite Station has the device and Satellite Station transfer	1. Blue corner aligned with the back corner of the Touchscreen	2. White adhesive tabs provide a tight fit on the Touchscreen
B. The back of the Satellite Station has the crank and handle	3. Slit provides access to crank and handle	4. Drape covers the Satellite Station transfer

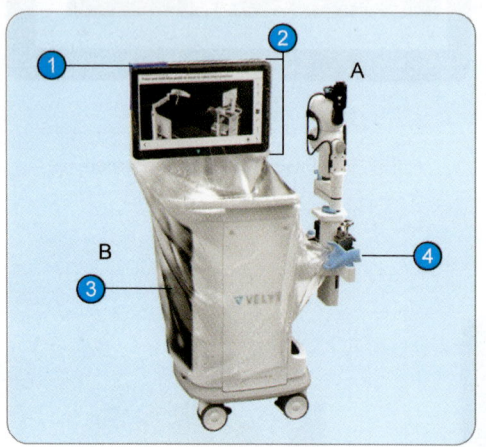

FIG. 9.9: Satellite Station.

Satellite Station Transfer Mechanism

Satellite Station Transfer mechanism supports the Robotic-Assisted Device Assembly during setup and aids in transferring the draped Robotic-Assisted Device assembly onto or off the bedrail. Between procedures, the Robotic-Assisted Device Assembly is stored on the Satellite Station Transfer.

The VELYS™ Robotic-Assisted Device Assembly (Fig. 9.10)

This includes:
- Robotic-assisted device (A)
- *Holding arm*: For vertical and horizontal movements (B)

The Robotic-Assisted Device has three rotational degrees of freedom, which enables it to position the PROCUT Saw Blade within any resection plane as desired during knee arthroplasty.

The Robotic-Assisted Device and Holding Arm are covered by a sterile drape **(Fig. 9.11)** for the entire surgical procedure. Prior to the resections, the draped Robotic-Assisted Device and Holding Arm are transferred from the Satellite Station to the bedrail.

CHAPTER 9: VELYS Robotic System

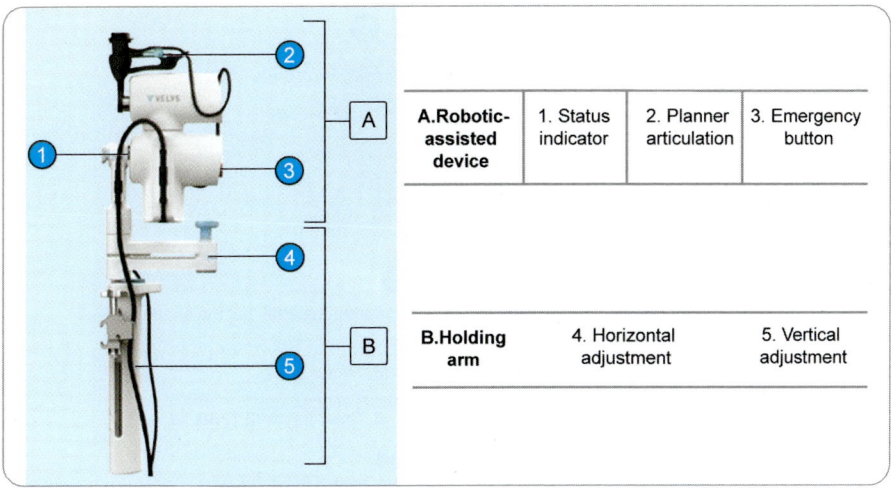

A	A. Robotic-assisted device	1. Status indicator	2. Planner articulation	3. Emergency button
B	B. Holding arm	4. Horizontal adjustment	5. Vertical adjustment	

FIG. 9.10: VELYS™ Robotic-Assisted device with the Holding Arm.

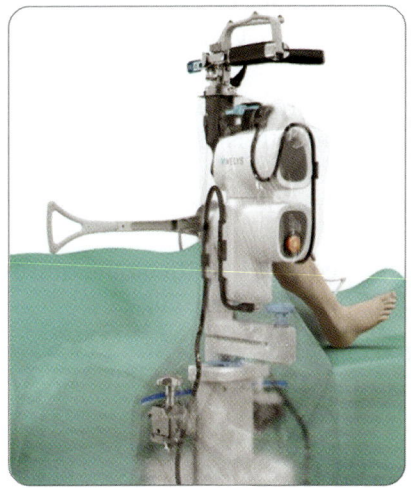

Note:
- *Status indicator on Robotic Device*: This is a color indicator that indicates the status of machine readiness during surgery; it also detects obstacles, if any.
- *Planar articulation*: Aids attachment of the saw.

FIG. 9.11: The Robotic-Assisted Device and Holding Arm covered by a sterile drape.

■ VELYS™ SINGLE USE INSTRUMENTS

Array Set: Knee

The arrays allow the system to identify and track the individual position of system components and the patient's bones. There are five types of arrays in one sterile pack **(Fig. 9.12)**, which are as underneath:

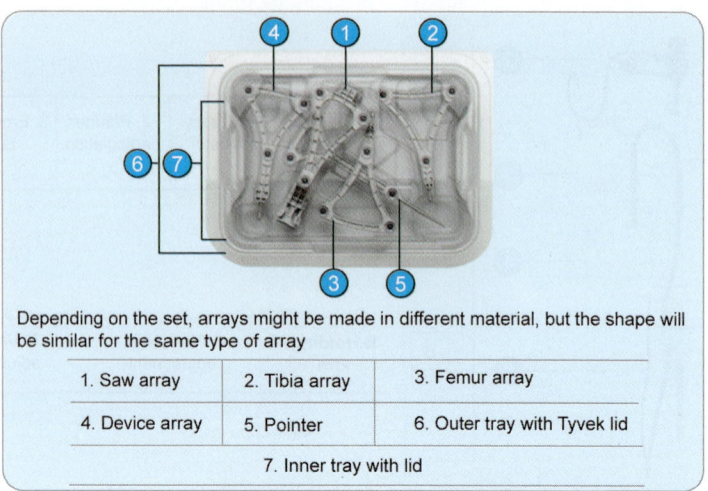

FIG. 9.12: The Array Set (Knee).

1. The Saw Array is used to track the Saw during resections.
2. The Device Array is used to track the Robotic-Assisted Device location and position.
3. The pointer is used to acquire anatomical landmarks on the patient's bones and to verify resected planes. It is also used to perform system checks and calibrations.
4. The Bone Arrays are fixed to the bones via the Array Drill Pins and the Array clamps.
5. The Femur Array is marked with FEMUR on the convex edge. The Tibia Array is marked with "TIBIA" on the concave edge.

Method of sterilization: Gamma rays

PROCUT Saw Blade

The PROCUT Saw Blade **(Fig. 9.13)** is system-specific. This robust 2 mm thick blade effortlessly cuts even the most sclerotic bones. The Saw Blade Cover, provided with the Saw Blade, protects the user from the sharp tip of the blade when the Saw Blade is not in use.

Method of sterilization: Gamma rays.

Array Drill Pins

The VELYS™ single-use array drill pins **(Fig. 9.14)** of 4 mm in diameter have the thinnest profile in the industry, which are used for any robot. This minimizes the available in different lengths (100, 125, and 175 mm) to accommodate femoral or tibial use and variations in patient anatomy or body mass index (BMI).

Method of sterilization: Gamma rays.

CHAPTER 9: VELYS Robotic System

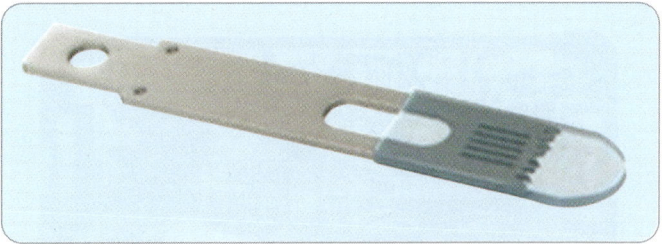

FIG. 9.13: PROCUT Saw Blade.

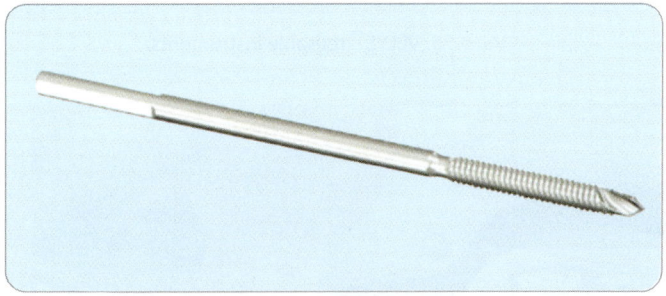

FIG. 9.14: Array Drill Pins.

Sterile Drapes

The Robotic-Assisted Device and Satellite Station are non-sterile and must be draped with system-specific sterile drapes before they are moved to the sterile field.

Method of sterilization: Ethylene Oxide (EO).

VELYS™ REUSABLE INSTRUMENTS (FIG. 9.15)

This includes all the reusable system-specific instruments like:
- The Saw Handpiece
- Array Clamp for Femur and Tibia
- Saw Interface (right and left)
- ATTUNE Lug Drill
- Caliper
- Tensor Spacer (5 and 10 mm)
- CAS Ligament Tensor (Size 2, Size 4)
- CAS Ligament Tensor Handle

VELYS™ LIGAMENT SENSOR TENSOR

Soft tissue balancing is a critical but often overlooked step in total knee arthroplasty (TKA). It is well accepted that soft tissue imbalance and bony malalignment in TKA lead to malfunction and failure. Studies have documented an incidence of

CHAPTER 9: VELYS Robotic System

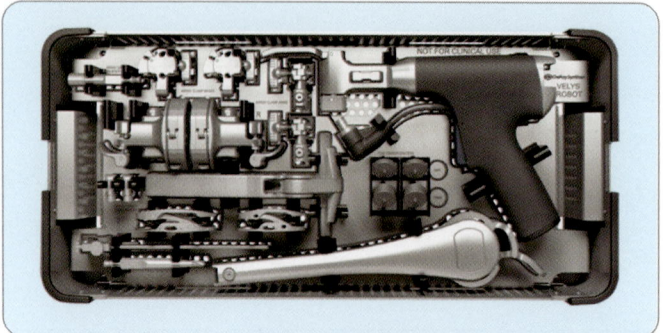

FIG. 9.15: VELYS™ reusable instruments.

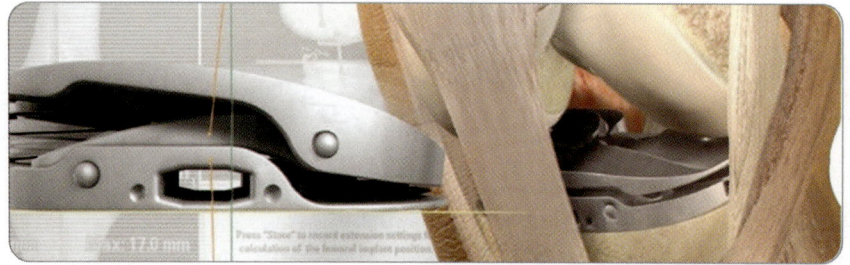

FIG. 9.16: VELYS™ Ligament Sensor Tensor.

revision for instability from 10 to 29%. It is important to consider, however, that although the general principles of ligament balancing are understood, there are still technical issues as well as different balancing philosophies that can affect the results.

The purpose of the VELYS™ Ligament Tensor **(Fig. 9.16)** is to achieve optimal alignment and balanced kinematics during robotically navigated TKA. The Tensor allows the ligament structures of the knee capsule to be equally tensioned, thereby facilitating reading of medial and lateral ligament laxity/tightness both in flexion and extension. This can only be used in the TIBIA FIRST technique of VELYS™.

■ VELYS™ GRAPHICAL USER INTERFACE

VELYS™ has the most user-friendly GUI. At each step the screen guides actions to perform to get ahead in plan.

Each screen has four parts, as presented below **(Fig. 9.17)**. Users can interact with the Desk and the Footer to move back and forth in the planning of surgery.

The Header and the Array Status Bar indicate the status of the system; they help with troubleshooting just by indicating the issue.

CHAPTER 9: VELYS Robotic System 97

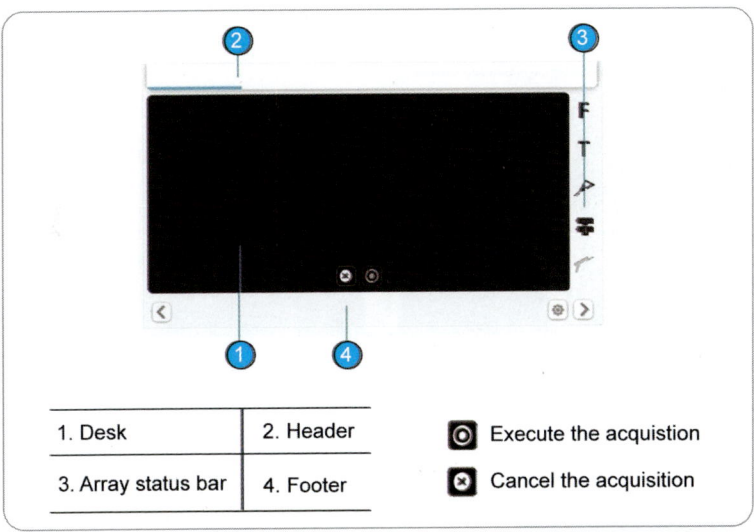

FIG. 9.17: VELYS™ Screen and Graphical User Interface.

ACCUBALANCE™ Graph Recording with Trial Implants

The super speedy ACCUBALANCE™ graph **(Fig. 9.18)** provides valuable insights such as:
- Type of femur component
- Size
- Insert thickness
- Refreshing the screen for repeat data
- Ligament balance with trial implants

Bring the leg into full extension and full flexion. Assess the final knee ROM. The software will automatically record the maximum extension and flexion for documentation in the case report. The red lines in the ligament balance graph **(Fig. 9.19)** indicate ligament tightness, while white represents adequate/lax ligaments.

▮ SETTING UP THE VELYS™ SYSTEM FOR CASE

As VELYS™ is an imageless robotic system, it does not need patients to undergo CT- and related radiation. One can plan surgery without any additional tests other than what we are usually doing to plan a TKR.

VELYS™ robot is set up for surgery during patient positioning, draping, and is ready for use before the incision takes place. This entire setup takes roughly 8–10 minutes before incision, and the best part is none of these setups interfere with routine surgical steps, so no additional time is needed than what we do manually. Also, in the VELYS™ system, multiple surgeon accounts can be created, which store surgeon-specific case data that is password protected for privacy.

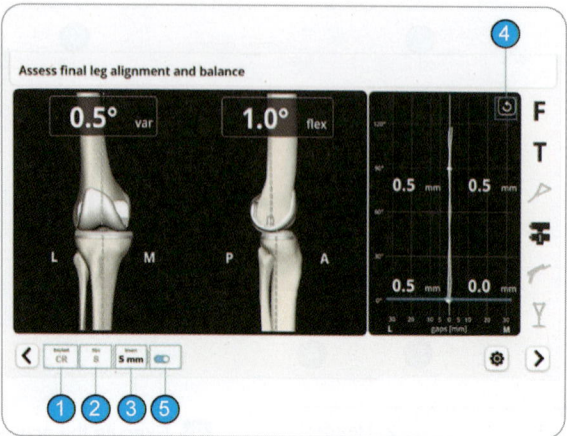

FIG. 9.18: ACCUBALANCE™ Graph.

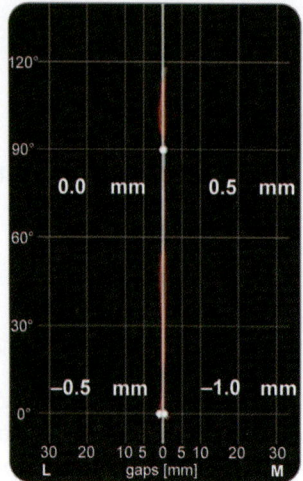

FIG. 9.19: Ligament Balance Graph.

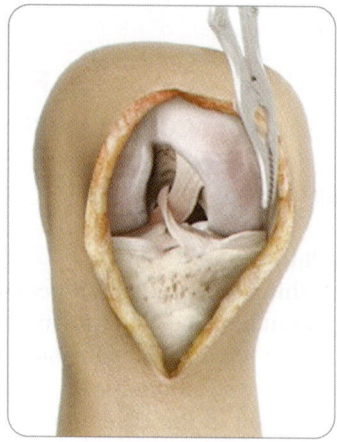

FIG. 9.20: Surgical exposure.

Incision, Exposure and Removal of Osteophytes

Surgical exposure **(Fig. 9.20)** can be made using the surgeon's preferred technique. This system allows removal of osteophytes and thus gives real data of ligament tightness/laxity and actual femur size basis true AP/ML. The advantage of the VELYS™ system is that it allows all four pins to be placed inside any type of incision, including minimally invasive surgical incisions.

Bony Landmark Acquisition

Checkpoints are small bone indentations created by the surgeon on the femur and tibia that are used as fixed reference points during the procedure to confirm that the Bone Arrays have not moved. They should be distinct, clear of soft tissue, and easily located.

The goal of this step is to acquire the anatomical landmarks that will be used by the system for computing the axis, planning resection depth, generating 3D models of the knee bones, and balancing the knee in flexion and extension, as well as throughout the ROM.

Position each checkpoint at a site where the bone will not be resected, e.g., below the anticipated tibial resection plane. Create each checkpoint cautiously with the appropriate instrument and into the cortical bone.

Tibial Checkpoint

Place the sharp tip of the Array Drill Pin on the tibial bone, below the tibial resection and adjacent to the tibial tubercle (TT) **(Fig. 9.21)**.

Femur Checkpoint

Repeat on the femoral bone in the region adjacent to the medial epicondyle **(Fig. 9.22)**.
- *Tip*: The checkpoints must be easily identifiable later during the procedure. Marking the checkpoints with a surgical pen will facilitate finding their location.

Array Drill Pin Placement

The 4 mm diameter single-use Array Drill Pins are available in different lengths to accommodate for variations in patient anatomy, BMI, or surgical techniques.
- *Tibial pin placement*: The Array Drill Pins are inserted three to four fingers below the incision and medial to the tibial crest **(Figs. 9.23A and B)**.
- Drill the Array Drill Pins perpendicular to the flat anteromedial tibial surface through the cortex to engage the posterolateral cortex. Drill through the center of the bone to avoid a purely cortical pin position. Care should be taken to avoid overpenetration of the posterolateral tibial cortex.

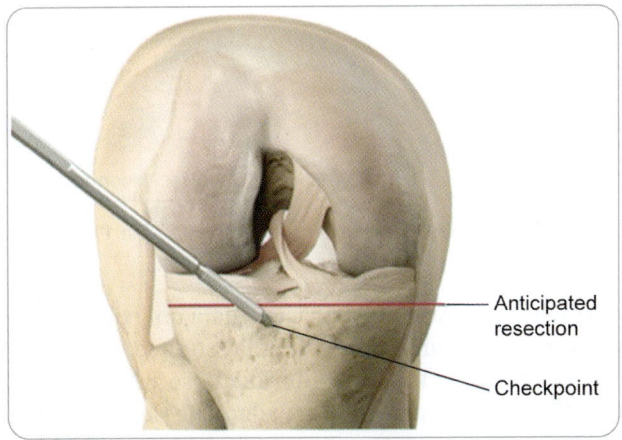

FIG. 9.21: Tibial checkpoint.

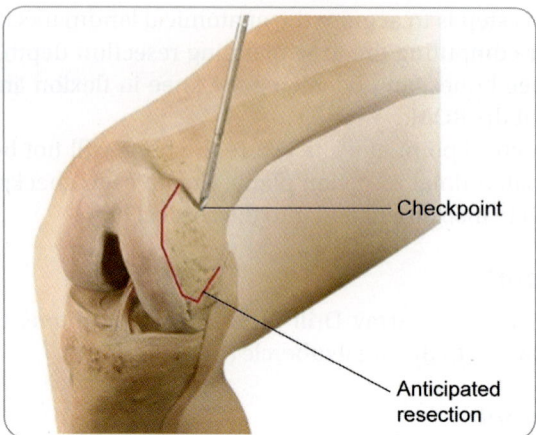

FIG. 9.22: Femur checkpoint.

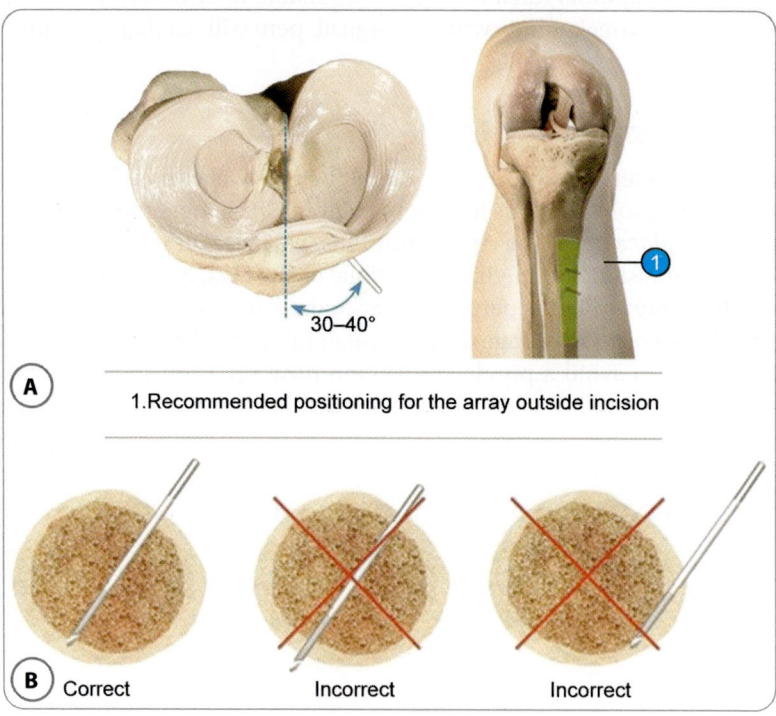

FIGS. 9.23A AND B: (A) Tibial Pin Placement and (B) Tibial Pin Placement.

For surgeons who want ACCUBALANCE™ data only till trial placement, they can put tibial pins 30–35 mm below the tibial surface, and tibial preparation can be done after removing the pins. But for those who want to get the final ACCUBALANCE™ graph, with implant adequate length must be planned considering keel placement.

When the tibial pins are placed distally, like shown in the figure, it even enables tibial preparation with stem extension. Also, we can have the final ACCUBALANCE™ graph after implanting with the stem in place.

Femur

Inside incision technique is recommended **(Fig. 9.24)**.

The Array Drill Pins are inserted proximal and anterior to the medial epicondyle, angling medially toward the camera at 30-50° relative to the sagittal plane.

Array Placement (Fig. 9.25)

Bone arrays are then attached by use of a pin wingnut, ensuring the visibility in both flexion and extension. Each Bone Array is fastened to the Array Clamp by

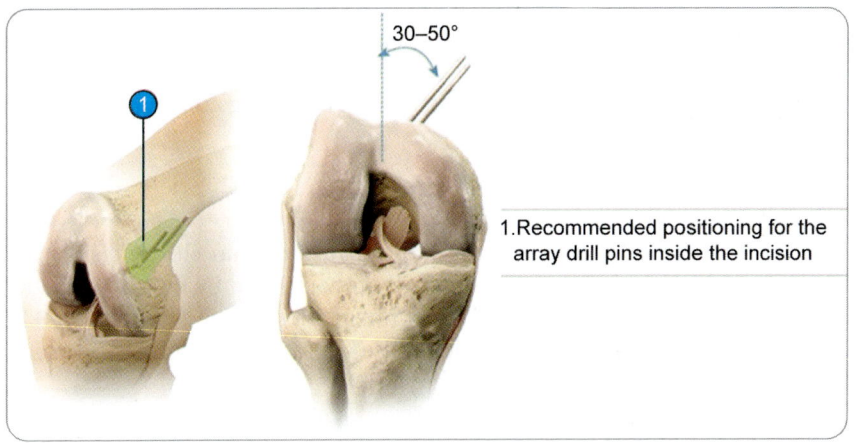

1. Recommended positioning for the array drill pins inside the incision

FIG. 9.24: Femur pin placement.

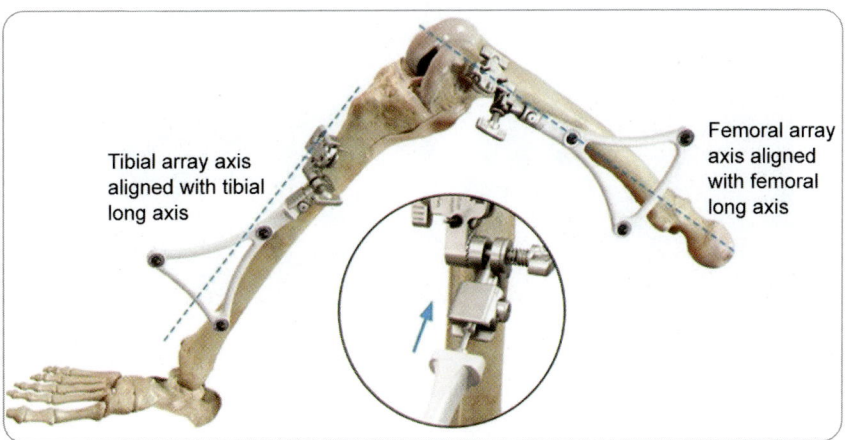

FIG. 9.25: Array Placement in Femur and Tibia.

pressing the button on the Array Clamp and engaging. VELYS™ has the simplest procedure for array placement. It takes less than a second to put the array in place.
- *Select the appropriate Bone Array*: Tibia Array or Femur Array.
- Align the Bone Array Tip with the Array Clamp Tip Hole.
- Press and hold the Array Clamp button. Insert the Bone Array Tip into the Array Clamp. Release the button and check that the Bone Array is rigidly fixed.
- The Bone Array should point away from the joint.
- Align the axis of the Bone Array parallel to the respective bone axis.

It is critical to have optimally placed and rigidly fixed Bone Arrays. Movement of the Arrays or loosening of the Array Drill Pins will compromise the accuracy of the system. Adjustments to the position of the Bone Arrays can be made:
- Prior to landmark registration
- Following the registration, but prior to bone resection.

This will require new registration of all landmarks for the bone where the Array was adjusted and new PROADJUST™ Surgical Planning. Adjustments are not permitted after the first bone resection: If Bone Array movement occurs, the reference frame becomes inaccurate. The Robotic-Assisted procedure must be aborted, and the procedure must be completed using conventional manual instruments.

Camera Adjustment

Adjust the Camera orientation so the Bone Arrays remain clearly visible at all likely leg positions during the procedure. This is achieved by matching both the alignment and diameter of the blue and white circles on the Screen **(Fig. 9.26)**. The blue circle defines the surgical field for the operative knee joint to be used for the robotic procedure.

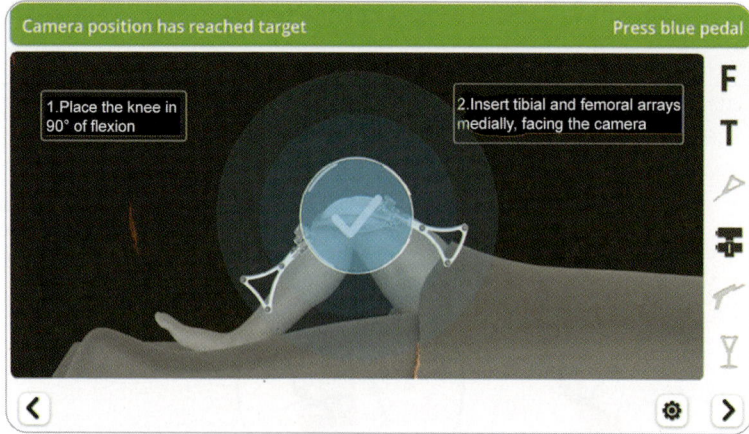

FIG. 9.26: Camera Position and Orientation seen on the Screen.

Check the visibility of the Bone Arrays in both flexion and extension. Ensure the two Bone Arrays always remain visible through a full knee ROM, i.e., the blue circle remains continuously visible on the screen. Adjust the Camera orientation and position as required to satisfy this condition before proceeding.

Landmarks Acquisition

The goal of this step is to acquire the anatomical landmarks and axes which will be used by the system for surgical planning.

Careful acquisition of landmarks is essential for the system to assess the joint, plan, implant position, balance, and alignment, and execute accurately. Small anatomical defects or protruding osteophytes that are not representative should not be acquired, as they may falsely represent the landmark needed.

In VELYS™ software, one needs to capture below mentioned 12 bony landmarks to generate a 3D joint image. This real-time, speedy registration takes only about 4 minutes, which is the quickest comparing any robotic system available for knee arthroplasty.

Computing Mechanical Axis using Bony Landmarks (Table 9.3)

- *Femoral center acquisition (**Figs. 9.27A and B**)*:
    - *Tip*: Circumduction of the hip in small to large circles
    - *Outcome*: Calculates the proximal extent of the femoral mechanical axis, which is the femoral head center
    - *What may go wrong*: Any movement of the pelvis, or the Camera, during acquisition will result in inaccurate calculation of the Femoral Head Center. This is most likely in patients with a high BMI or a stiff hip. Options include:
        - Have the assistant secure the pelvis by applying pressure to one or both ASIS.
        - Temporary release of the lateral side leg support to allow free motion of the leg.
        - Decrease the arc of motion of the leg not to move the pelvis
- *Tibial mechanical axis*: Distal
  The most prominent points of the malleoli can usually be located by palpation before acquiring the landmarks. Place the tip of the Pointer on the most

TABLE 9.3: Computing mechanical axis using bony landmarks.		
Mechanical axis	**Axis point**	**Landmark**
Femoral	Proximal	Femoral head center—acquired by hip circumduction
	Distal	Femoral knee center—acquired by single-point registration
Tibial	Proximal	Tibial knee center—acquired by single-point registration
	Distal	Midpoint of the malleoli—calculated following single-point registration of the medial and lateral malleoli

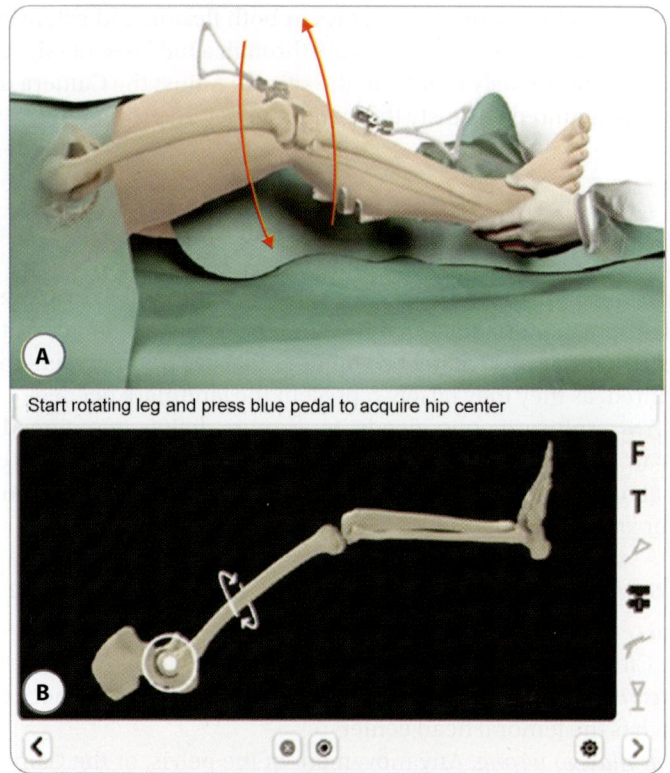

FIGS. 9.27A AND B: Femoral center acquisition.

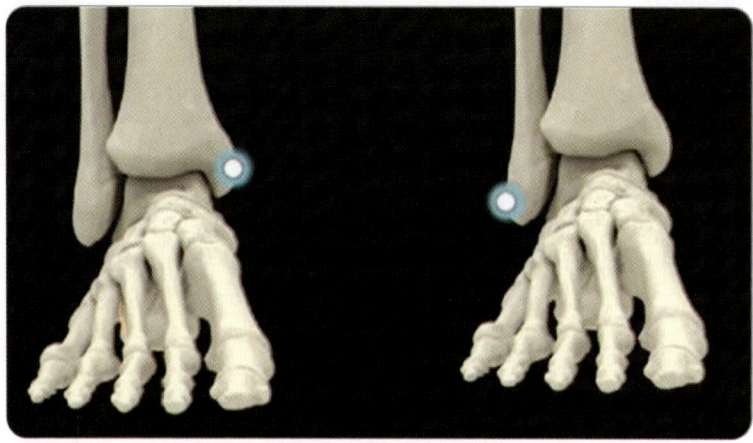

FIG. 9.28: Tibial Mechanical Axis: Distal.

prominent medial point of the medial malleolus **(Fig. 9.28)**. This is not the tip of the malleolus, but its most prominent protuberance.
- *Tip*: These points should be precisely collected in both the proximal-distal and anterior-posterior directions for the system to accurately calculate

tibial slope. Don't acquire malleoli over a thick wrap. Care should be taken for patients with severe ankle deformity, where the malleoli may not represent accurate landmarks for defining the tibial mechanical axis.
- *Outcome*: Calculates the distal extent of the tibial mechanical axis by computing the midpoint from the medial and lateral malleoli **(Fig. 9.29)**.
- *What may go wrong*: A thick wrap around the ankle may give a false feel of the malleoli. The wrong point of acquisition may lead to the wrong tibial axis, thus wrong flexion in ROM.

- *Tibial knee center*:
  - *Tip*: This point will define the intersection of the midcoronal and midsagittal planes of the tibia (center of the proximal tibia), to be precise ACL footprint.
  - Outcome: This point should be collected in the anterior-posterior direction for the system to accurately calculate tibial slope **(Fig. 9.30)**.
  - What may go wrong: Inaccuracy in this point may give the wrong tibial slope, affecting flexion space.

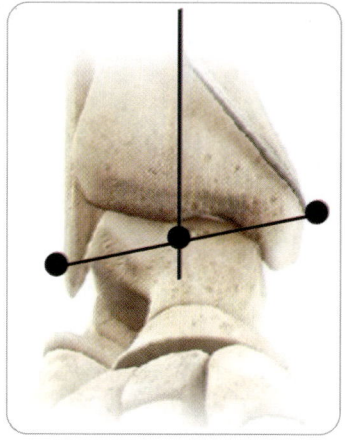

FIG. 9.29: Tibial Mechanical Axis.

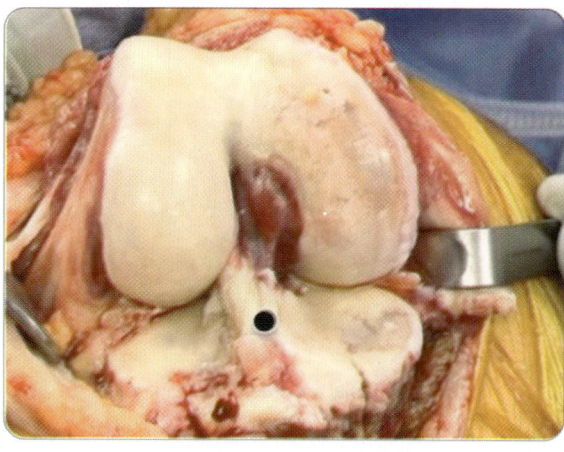

FIG. 9.30: Tibial knee center.

- *Tibial plateau*: The goal of the acquisition of a single point on each plateau (medial and lateral) is to define the tibial resection level **(Fig. 9.31)**.

  Each point should be representative of resection reference the surgeon desires on each side. The initial resection height is measured from the highest of these two points **(Fig. 9.32)**. The default value for this height is 9 mm.
  - *Tip*: Medial plateau—take a point at the lowest articulating point.
  - *Lateral plateau*: Take a point at the highest articulating point.
  - *Outcome*: Set resection depth medially and laterally.
  - *What may go wrong*: In some cases, e.g., cartilage or bone wear, the highest point found and acquired on the lateral plateau might be lower than the native highest point. This will result in over-resection of the proximal tibia. In this case, during PROADJUST™ Surgical Planning, the surgeon may need to reduce the resection depth to avoid over-resection.

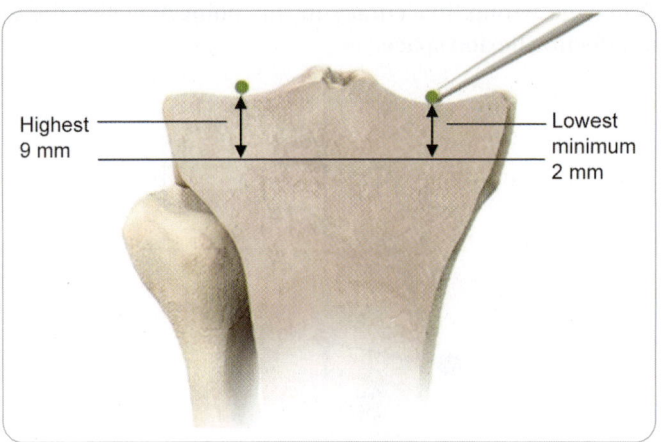

FIG. 9.31: Tibial resection level.

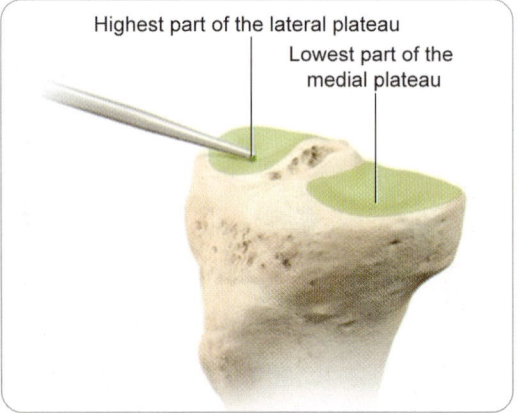

FIG. 9.32: Medial and lateral plateau points.

- *Tibial sagittal axis*:
  - *Tip*: It is important that this direction is set in neutral rotation, through the center of the tibia. Failure to do so can result in inaccuracies both in the sagittal and coronal planes when defining the tibial resection.
  - Aligning with the posterior cruciate ligament (PCL) insertion and medial one-third TT sagittal alignment is less critical.
  - *Outcome*: The acquisition of the tibial sagittal axis will define the direction of the sagittal plane **(Fig. 9.33)**.
  - *What may go wrong*: The tibial slope is calculated within the sagittal plane. Thus, while this sagittal axis acquisition does not set the tibial slope directly, it will influence the slope indirectly by changing the sagittal plane position. Internal or external rotation will result in an oblique slope as shown in the image **(Figs. 9.34A and B)**.
- *Femur knee center*:
  - *Tip*: Landmark, just anterior to the apex of the notch **(Fig. 9.35)**.
  - *Outcome*: calculates the distal extent of the femoral mechanical axis.
  - *What may go wrong*: An incorrect point may affect the extension space.
- *Whiteside's line [anteroposterior (AP) axis]*:
  - *Tip*: Place the pointer along Whiteside's line—the line created by connecting the points in the deepest part of the trochlea groove **(Figs. 9.36A and B)**.
  - *Outcome*: Additional femoral rotational axis reference
  - *What may go wrong*: May affect the data showing rotation with respect to the posterior condylar axis (PCA).
- *Distal femoral condyles (DFC)*: DFC registration will identify the most distal point of the medial and lateral femoral condyles **(Figs. 9.37A and B)**. These points are used for measuring the distal resection depth. This is achieved by mapping the surface of both distal condyles with the Pointer. The software will then automatically determine the most distal point of each condyle.
  - *Tip*: Place the probe on the distal femoral joint surface first and then move the pointer as if it is "painting." Be sure to capture the distal-most point. Avoid taking any point in the air.

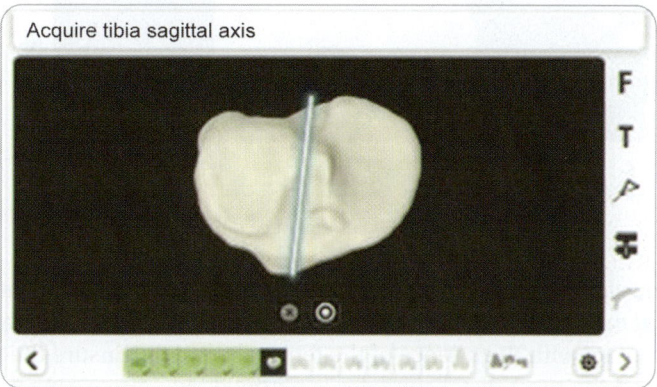

FIG. 9.33: Tibial sagittal axis.

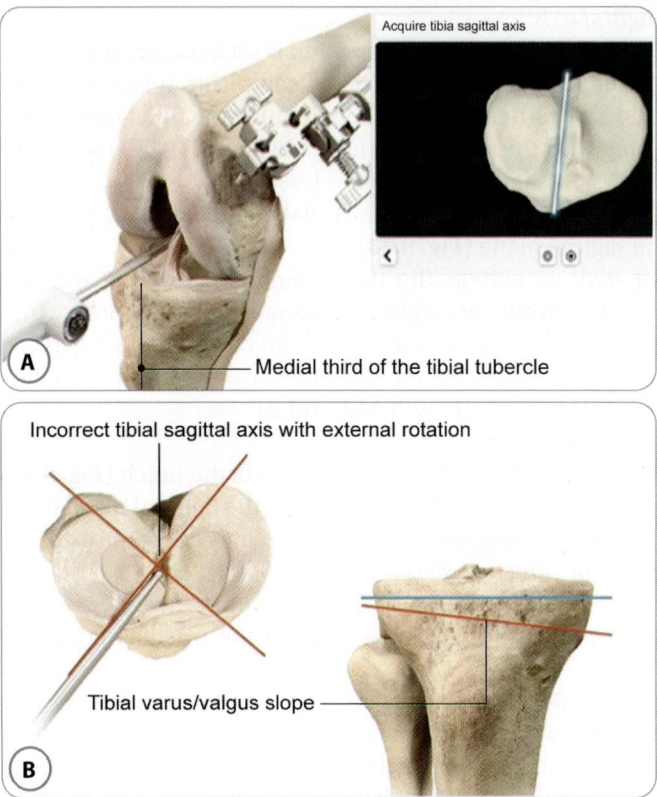

FIGS. 9.34A AND B: The tibial slope.

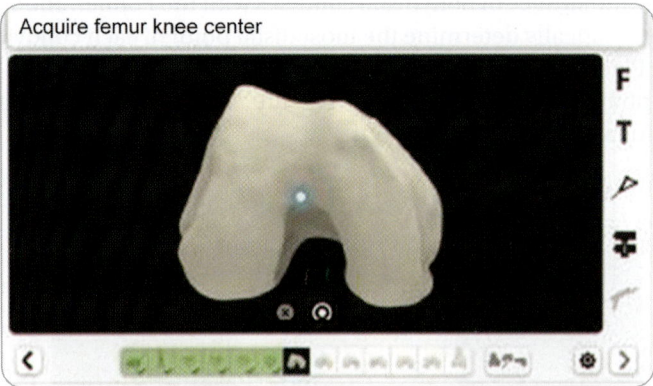

FIG. 9.35: Femur knee center.

- *Outcome*: Establishes point for resection depth medially and laterally.
- *What may go wrong*: While mapping, ensure the Pointer tip is always kept in contact with the surface of the femoral condyle. Ensure the entire area around the most distal condyles is mapped. Avoid mapping osteophytes, which may protrude from the condyles.

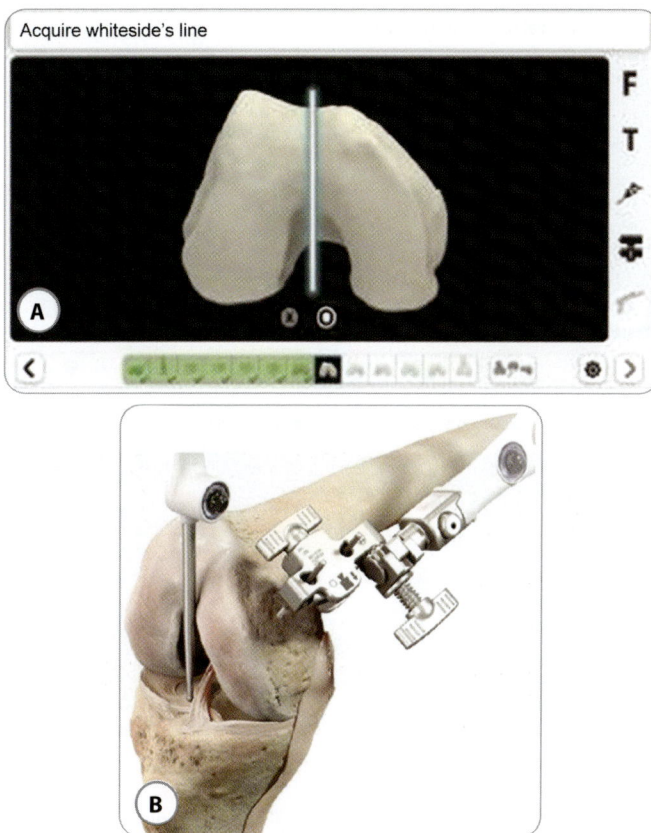

FIGS. 9.36A AND B: Whiteside's line (anteroposterior axis).

Mapping the wrong/not most prominent point will give wrong resection DFC medial and lateral values.

Too much medial or too much lateral point will give wrong mediolateral values, computing either an undersized or an oversized femur size.

- *Posterior femoral condyles* **(Figs. 9.38A and B)**:
  - *Tip*: Place the probe on the posterior femoral joint surface first and then move the pointer as if it is "painting." Use caution to avoid levering off the femur. Use the long axis of the femur as a reference.
  - *Outcome*: Establishes point for resection depth for medial and lateral sides posteriorly, PCA identification.
  - *What may go wrong*: Mapping the wrong/posterior point will give wrong posterior resection values medially and laterally.

Too many inferior or inaccurate posterior points will give wrong AP values, resulting in either an undersized or an oversized femur size.

- *Anterior cortex*: The anterior cortex registration **(Fig. 9.39)** will be used to:
  - Calculate the femoral implant size.
  - Determine the initial AP position of the femoral implant.
  - Quantify the position of the implant anterior flange relative to the anterior cortex (notching or gap).

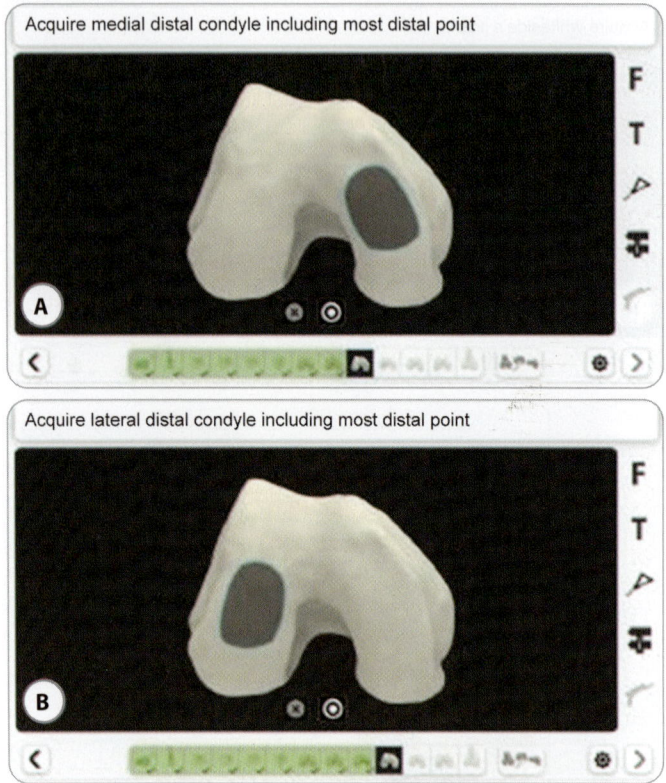

FIGS. 9.37A AND B: Distal femoral condyle registration.

- *Tip*: Start proximal to your normal stylus position by 50% of the length. Move distally with pace and move the pointer as if splitting the lateral condyle. Clear or incise soft tissue/osteophytes prior to capturing.
- *Outcome*: Establishes point for anterior resection, sizing, and notch prevention.
- *What may go wrong*: Inaccurate point acquisition will lead to wrong AP, improper femoral size, and may notch while taking anterior resection.

Confirmation of Acquired Landmarks

The confirmation screen displays the landmarks that have been extracted from the five "painted" areas to allow a visual check of each acquired landmark [represented on screen by a green dot outlined in white **(Fig. 9.40)**]. The five points can be checked in any order.

The system will measure the "offset," which is the difference in position between:
- The tip of the pointer.
- The point determined by the system during acquisition (green dot) in the proximal-distal direction for the posterior condyles and in the anterior-posterior direction for the posterior condyles and anterior cortex.

CHAPTER 9: VELYS Robotic System

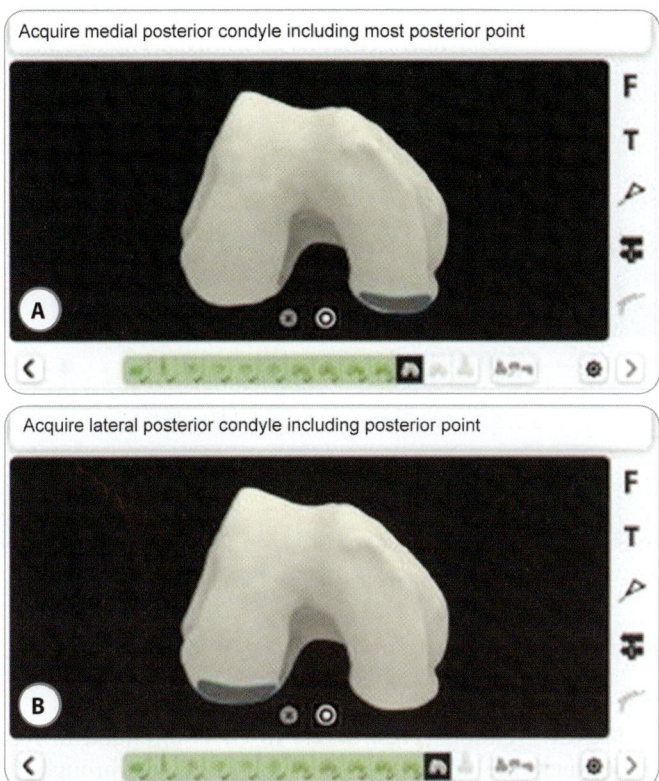

FIGS. 9.38A AND B: Posterior femoral condyles registration.

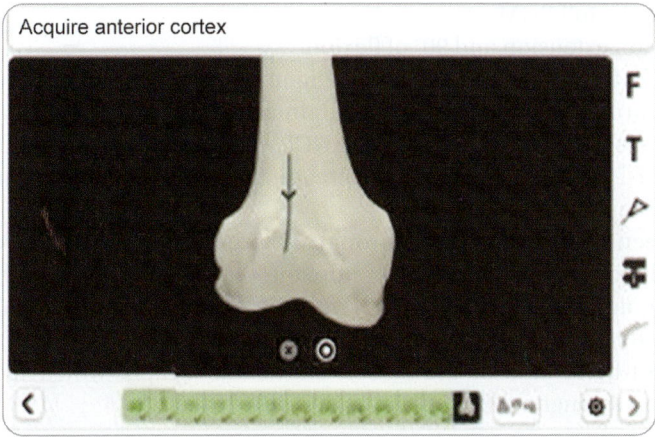

FIG. 9.39: Anterior cortex registration.

Repeat Landmark Acquisition

If the surgeon is not satisfied with the confirmation of landmarks, repeating the acquisition of the relevant landmarks before proceeding to the next step is super quick and one need not retake all other landmarks **(Fig. 9.41)**. That is what makes the system highly efficient and speedy.

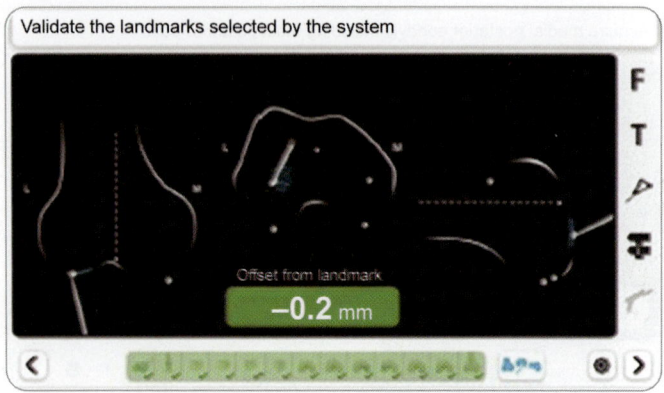

FIG. 9.40: Confirmation of acquired landmarks.

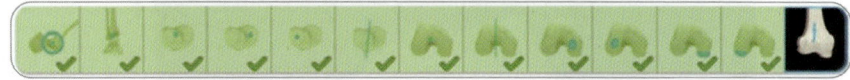

FIG. 9.41: Repeat landmark acquisition.

Initial Leg Alignment and ACCUBALANCE™ Graph Recording

The ACCUBALANCE™ Graph **(Figs. 9.42A to C)** is intended to represent the relationship between the tibial and femoral implants through flexion and extension with the soft tissues in the intended tension.

There are two possible options for recording the graph:
1. Through the full ROM, or
2. Only in full extension and 90° of flexion

The goal of this step is to assess leg alignment and knee balance. Combined with the information acquired during landmarks acquisition, the data recorded during this step creates the ACCUBALANCE™ Graph, which is modified during PROADJUST™ Surgical Planning to create the desired final alignment and balance of the knee.

The screen shows the current coronal and sagittal alignment [hip knee ankle (HKA) angle] of the knee, the type of implant, the calculated size of the femoral component, and the insert thickness (which is by default 5 mm initially). These can be adjusted with a corresponding change in the ACCUBALANCE™ Graph.

The right-hand side of the screen shows the Graph, which displays the expected gap throughout the ROM.

Initial PROADJUST™ Surgical Planning (Fig. 9.43)

The initial implant size and position are determined automatically based on the landmarks acquired and the parameters set by the surgeon in the surgical profile. Clinical judgment is required to determine the appropriate resection amount on both distal condyles, especially in cases of wear or severe deformity. Adjust the distal femoral resection and/or the coronal alignment of the resection as required.

CHAPTER 9: VELYS Robotic System

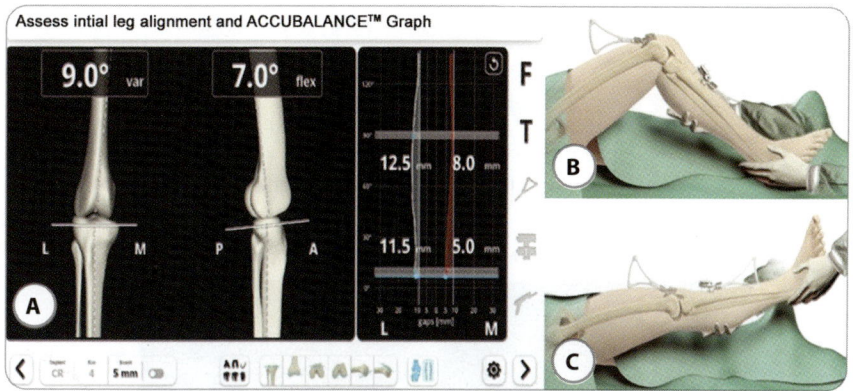

FIGS. 9.42A TO C: ACCUBALANCE™ Graph.

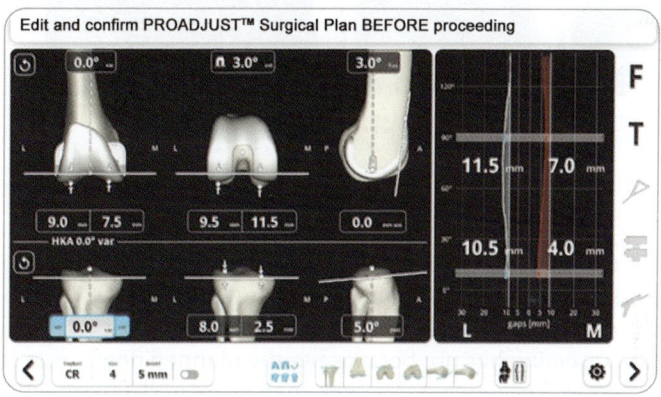

FIG. 9.43: PROADJUST™ surgical planning.

Performing Resections

Each resection will be performed in two steps:
1. Position the leg and retractors, then move the Robotic-Assisted Device to the precise resection plane.
2. Resection of the bone.
   The system will display a specific screen for each step **(Fig. 9.44)**.

The cuts performed by the system are as discussed here:
- Distal femur resection
- Proximal tibial resection
- Anterior femur resection
- Posterior femur resection
- Anterior chamfer and posterior chamfer
   In case of posterior-stabilized (PS) knee surgery, a box cut needs to be taken manually.

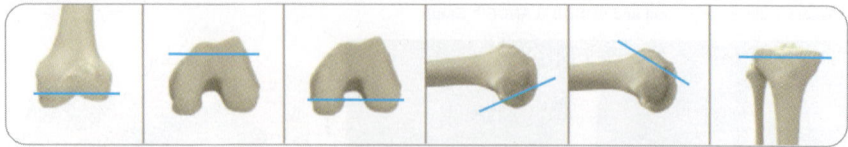

FIGS. 9.44: Resection of the bone markers.

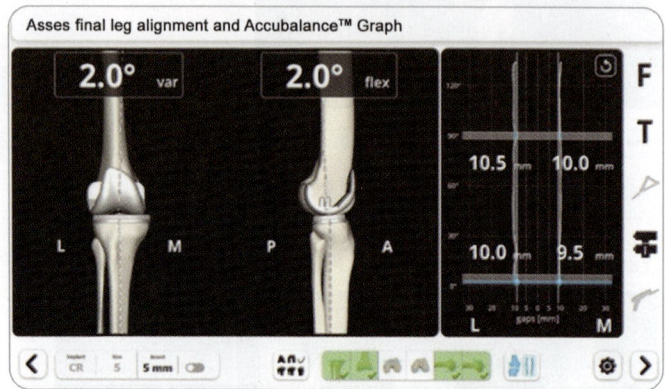

FIGS. 9.45: Final leg assessment.

After each cut, the pointer array helps in verifying the cut surface for accuracy of planned resection/deviation from resection depth, if any. Deviation of cuts more than 1mm requires re-touch of the cut surface.

In case the resection has not been as per the planned depth, one can retouch the cut in fractions of seconds. Moreover, increasing or decreasing the resection or femoral rotation, flexion, or extension of the femoral component and slope takes only a few seconds, and the resection plane gets adjusted accordingly.

One can plan resections in any order. For the femur-first technique, the femur needs to be finished first; however, for the tibia-first technique, the tibial cut is necessary for using the ligament tensioner device known as the sensor tensor. One may also use a hybrid method of resection if desired.

In my opinion, VELYS™ Sensor Tensor is an immensely helpful tool in planning the flexion extension gap after the tibial cut.

Final Leg Assessment

In the last step, the final leg alignment and balance of the knee in flexion and extension. The above image shows ligament balance without the trial implants **(Fig. 9.45)**.

The screen has an option to show the ligament balance with the trial implant as well **(Fig. 9.46)**.

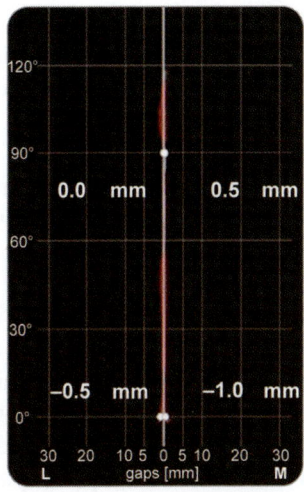

FIGS. 9.46: Ligament balance gaps.

CONVENTIONAL VERSUS ROBOTIC TKR (VELYS™)

- *Exposure*: The approach remains the same. Any type of incision is well accepted with VELYS™. In fact, the incision can be smaller than in manual surgery, as VELYS™ functions effectively even with Minimally Invasive Surgical (MIS) incisions
- *Additional time for VELYS™ compared to manual TKR*:
    - *Pin placement*: 1–2 minutes.
    - *Registration*: 2–3 minutes (Repeat registration, if needed, add 1 minute)
    - *Initial leg assessment*: 1 minute.
    - *Planning on ProAdjust*: It may take around 10 minutes. In the first 15–20 cases, planning may take longer. However, with experience, it reduces to 3–4 minutes.
    - *Resection of tibia and femur*: 5–7 minutes. *Recuts (if needed)*: Additional 1–2 minutes
    - *Final leg assessment*: 1 minute.
- *Time efficiency with experience*: Initially, VELYS™-specific steps add 15–25 minutes to your routine TKR time. However, after 20–25 cases, the procedure becomes time-neutral. Beyond 50 cases, VELYS™ can actually save time due to:
    - Elimination of jig assembly at each step.
    - Faster decision-making with real-time system data.
    - Simplified and precise fine-tuning of ligament balance, even in complex cases.

VELYS™ ROBOTIC ASSISTED SYSTEM ADVANTAGES

VELYS™ System is well adapted for:

- CR as well as PS cases. The Attune Implant design and the ease of balancing with VELYS™ have led many PS surgeons to transition to CR.
- Femur first or tibia first or hybrid workflow can be used; however, tibia first has the advantage of using the Sensor Tensor Device for balancing
- The system works exclusively with the ATTUNE™ Knee System, which has been used by over 1 million patients worldwide and is designed to deliver a greater ROM and faster recovery, and greater functional outcomes. Attune has the advantage of a rotating platform in both CR and PS, which no other system offers.
    - Bilateral knee replacement is easier and more efficient with the VELYS™ Robotic System. Its precise planning, real-time data, and ease of adjustments streamline the procedure, reducing surgical time while ensuring optimal alignment and balance for both knees.
    - No CT required, no radiation exposure or added cost burden to patients.
    - VELYS™ features two screens, a unique capability not offered by any other system. The Satellite Station screen can be used by the surgeon after draping and placing it in the sterile field, eliminating the need for dependence on industry personnel for OR support.
    - Smallest footprint amongst all the other available robots for knee arthroplasty helps in optimization of OT space and OR efficiency.
    - Saw-based cutting gives speed to the overall surgery, just like manual one, with its robust 2 mm thick blade.
    - Advanced Pure Sight hydrophobic optical technology and high-speed camera effectively tracks all movements of the knee and adjust the cut plane accordingly.
    - VELYS™ Array tracker use is the easiest of compared to any other robotic system
    - Thin pin profiles (4 mm) and no additional jigs make it safe to use without risk of fracture track or impact won bone.
    - Cost of consumables is at par with any robotic system, and in fact, less in comparison to CT-based systems
    - The accuracy of femoral size, ligament balance, and user-friendly software make it a great choice for both budding and established orthopedic surgeons.
    - With repeated use, there is no increase in OR time compared to the surgeon's own manual surgery time. Beyond 50 cases, one is likely to cut down on OR time
    - The VELYS™ Robotic-Assisted Solution works exclusively with the ATTUNE™ Knee System, which is designed to deliver a greater ROM and faster recovery, and greater functional outcomes.

■ VELYS™ ROBOTIC ASSISTED SYSTEM DISADVANTAGES

- As of now, the VELYS™ system has only TKR software in it; THR and UKR software are yet to be launched.
- It cannot be transported from hospital to hospital

- The plan of surgery depends on the accuracy of bony landmarks, thus if one fails to take correct landmarks the whole plan can prove to be incorrect

Scan to learn more about VELYS™ Robotic Surgery: The Future of Precision, Accuracy, and Faster

CONCLUSION

VELYS™ stands true to its name, derived from velocity, i.e., speed.

Its user-friendly interface provides operational confidence to surgeons across all levels of experience and expertise.

It predicts femur size quite accurately. In case of medial laxity, it is surprising how quickly it gets picked up by the software even when the laxity is not visible to the naked eye. Planning with PROADJUST is super easy and super astonishing to see, and the use of femoral flex/extension or rotation in balancing the overall knee, which was never possible in manual surgery otherwise. It is the most user-friendly system available for knee replacement surgeries.

CHAPTER 10

CORI Robotic System

Ashish Phadnis, Pramod Bhor, Sawankumar Pawar, Gaurav Patel, Sachin Yashwant Kale, Neharika Tandon

INTRODUCTION

CORI™ Surgical System is an advanced, handheld robotics-assisted platform designed to enhance the precision and efficiency of joint arthroplasty procedures. CORI Robotic System is a semiactive handheld surgical robot developed by Smith and Nephew Ltd. This system integrates real-time personalized intraoperative feedback using handheld robotics image-free smart mapping to optimize patient-specific implant alignment and balance. The dimensions for CORI system as described below **(Table 10.1)**.
- *Robotic cart = 105 lbs (47.62 kgs)*
- *CORI console power rating = 175 VA*
- *Robotics cart power rating = 230 VA*

SHAPE AND ERGONOMIC DESIGN

Amongst all the floor mounted robots, CORI has a compact design hence integrates into the OR with minimal setup. Storage and maneuverability are easier causing quick room turnover and facility to facility portability.

CORI CONSOLE

Central to CORI™ Surgical System functionality is the Robotics Console, a compact and portable unit that integrates several key components **(Fig. 10.1)**.
- *Ergonomic handpiece*: This handheld device features burr designs that deliver twice the cutting volume, enabling faster bone preparation **(Fig. 10.2)**.

TABLE 10.1: Robotic dimensions and weight.

	Dimensions
CORI Robotic Cart + CORI Console (max)	698 mm (L) × 590 mm (W) × 1952 mm (H)
CORI Robotic Cart + CORI Console (min)	698 mm (L) × 590 mm (W) × 1813 mm (H)

CHAPTER 10: CORI Robotic System

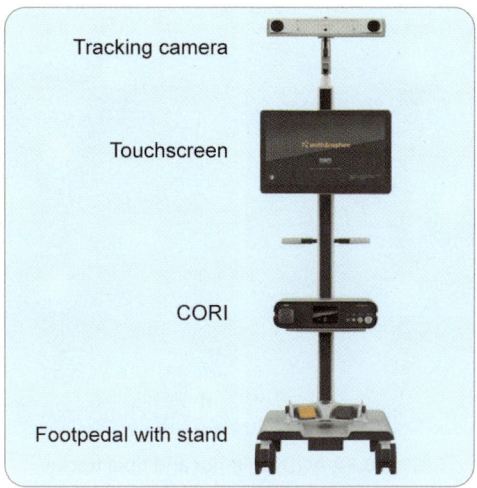

FIG. 10.1: CORI Console and its parts.

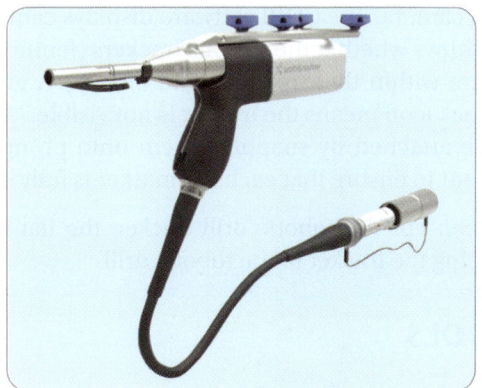

FIG. 10.2: Ergonomic handpiece.

- *ATRACSYS™ Advanced Tracking System*: A high-speed optical tracking camera that offers a 458% faster refresh rate, facilitating real-time navigation and precise instrument guidance during surgery.
- *Touchscreen tablet*: It provides an interactive interface for surgical planning and intraoperative adjustments, allowing surgeons to create and modify surgical plans directly in the operating room.
- *Foot pedal*: It allows surgeons to control certain system functions hands-free, enhancing workflow efficiency during procedures.

VISION SYSTEM AND MARKER SPECIFICATIONS

Vision system of the *real intelligence CORI* for knee arthroplasty primarily involves the tracking camera and the trackers that are attached to the patient's femur and tibia, as well as instruments like the point probe and robotic drill.

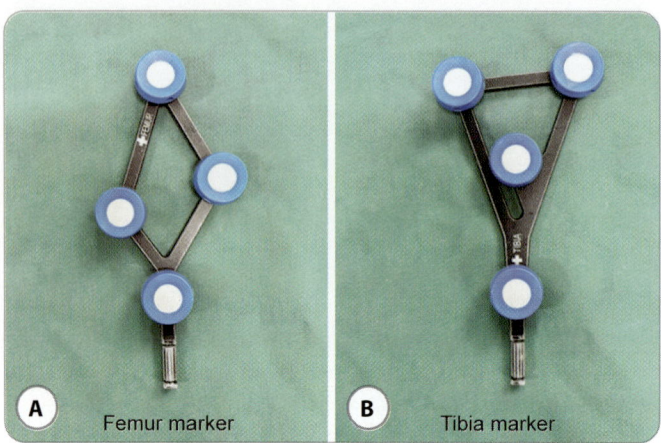

FIGS. 10.3A AND B: Femur and tibia tracker.

It is crucial to orient the flat markers on the femur tracker **(Figs. 10.3A and B)** toward the tracking camera. The CORI software displays camera view indicators on the screen that shows whether the various trackers (femur, tibia, point probe, and robotic drill) are within the camera's field of view. A green icon indicates visibility, while a black icon means the tracker is not visible.

Flat markers are attached by snapping them onto prongs located on each tracker. It is important to ensure that each flat marker is fully seated.

Timing of attachment: For the robotic drill tracker, the flat markers should be added before attaching the tracker to the robotic drill.

CUTTING TOOLS

Robotic Drill and Burs (Figs. 10.4A and B)

The robotic drill is a key component for bone removal and preparing fixation features.
- 6-mm bullet bur
- 6-mm chip breaker bullet bur
- 5-mm and 6-mm cylindrical bur

The selection of the bur depends on the implant type and the specific step in the procedure, such as preparing postholes for UKA implants or for specific cut guide techniques in total knee arthroplasty (TKA).

A robotic drill guard **(Fig. 10.5)** and robotic drill attachment is used with the robotic drill.

Different control modes for the robotic drill—exposure and speed, as well as an OFF (manual) mode. These modes affect how the bur interacts with the bone and the virtual model.

There are warnings associated with the robotic drill and burs including the risk of lacerations from sharp objects, potential for overheating and the need for

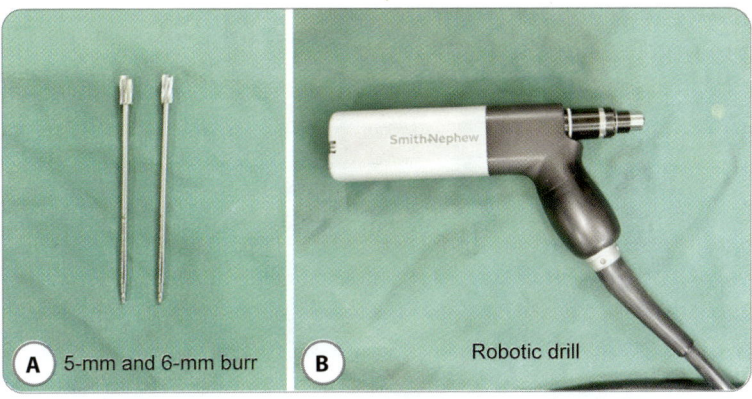

FIGS. 10.4A AND B: Burr and robotic drill.

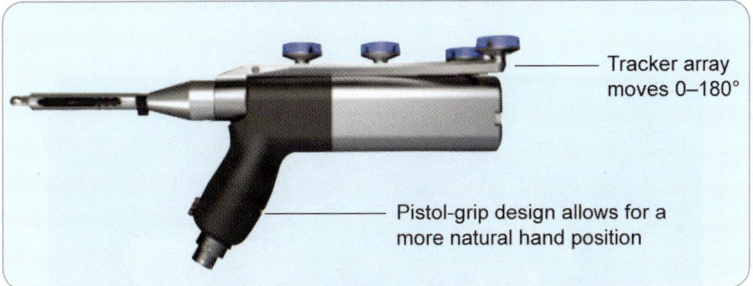

FIG. 10.5: Robotic drill with burr and trackers attached.

adequate irrigation and suction during use to prevent bone damage and prolong the attachment's life. Surgeons are also warned to use retractors to protect soft tissues and to avoid overcutting.

Saw Blades (Fig. 10.6)

While the robotic drill and burs are used for initial bone preparation and creating fixation features, saw blades are recommended for completing bulk bone removal based on the cut guides placed. The recommended saw blade thickness for TKA systems is 1.35 mm.

Cut Guides

Cut guides are used in conjunction with the robotic drill and subsequently with saw blades to achieve accurate bone cuts.

CORI supports various cut guide options for both the femur and tibia in TKA procedures, including "Bur All," "Distal Precision Burring," and "Robotics Distal Cut Guide" for the femur, and options like "Twin Peg" for the tibia **(Figs. 10.7A and B)**.

CHAPTER 10: CORI Robotic System

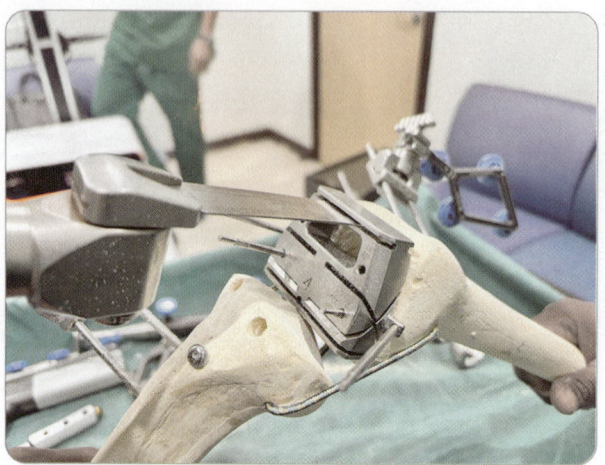

FIG. 10.6: Saw blade on bone saw model.

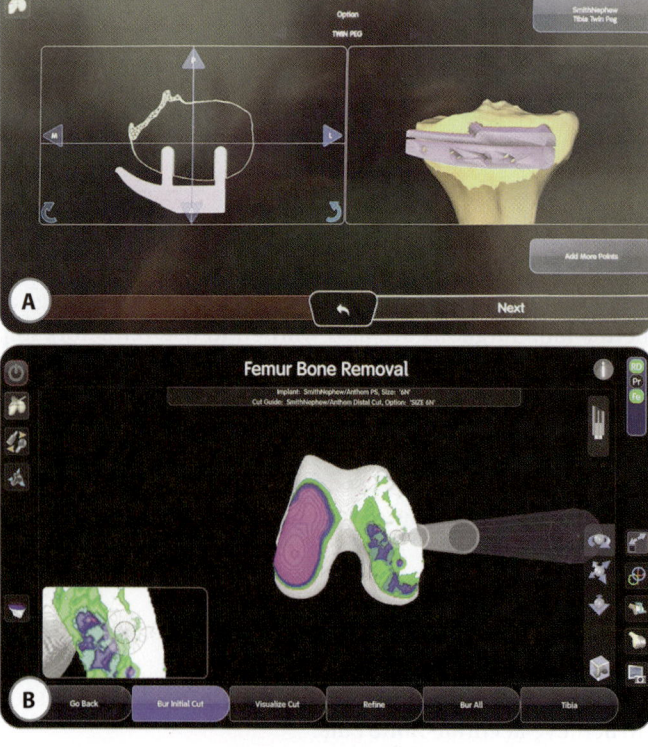

FIGS. 10.7A AND B: Cut guide for tibia and femur.

Point Probe (Fig. 10.8)

The point probe (ROB10017) is used for collecting landmark points on the bone surface during the free collection stages to characterize the patient's anatomy. While not a cutting tool, it is crucial for defining the surgical plan that guides bone removal.

A plane visualization tool can be attached to the point probe to visualize the planned cut planes during and after bone removal, allowing for comparison with the actual cut.

Rasp (Fig. 10.9)

A rasp is included in the robotics instruments tray. It may be needed to make fine adjustments to bone preparations completed with the robotic drill, particularly for squaring the tibial corner in unicondylar knee replacement (UKR) procedures and the box for the posterior cruciate ligament (PCL).

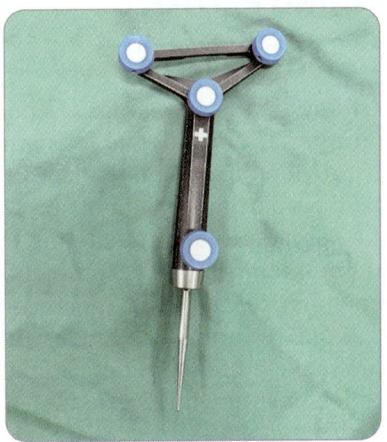

FIG. 10.8: Point probe.

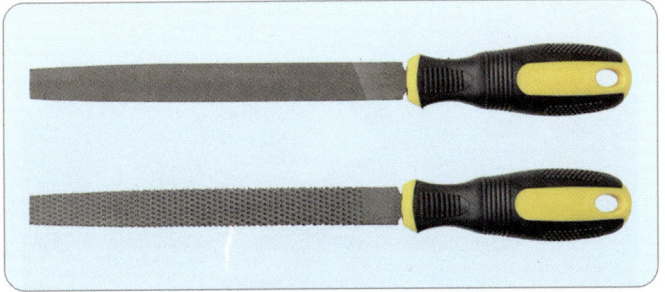

FIG. 10.9: Rasp.

CORI SOFTWARE

- Designed to be portable with a small OR footprint, the CORI Surgical System uses real intelligence software to offer broad capabilities and an expanding range of joint reconstruction indications—TKA, UKA, and revision TKA. Image-free smart mapping eliminates potential for image distortion caused by in situ components, with 3D joint models registering anatomy and bony defects after implant extraction.
- CORI Virtual Planner provides an interactive, fully functional software tool for surgeons to become familiar with creating a surgical plan on the CORI Surgical System.
- This on-demand tool is accessible anywhere, anytime through S + N Academy Online—an on-line accredited platform offering comprehensive educational materials, interactive courses, and valuable resources from world-class surgeons and opinion leaders on robotic-assisted surgery.

SURGICAL PLANNING PROTOCOL

Patient and System Setup (Fig. 10.10)

Proper setup of the CORI system is crucial for a smooth surgical workflow. The CORI graphical user interface is designed for surgeons to simply operate during planning and provide visual guidance during operation. After positioning the device and preparing the patient, apply sterile curtains on the monitor. This allows the surgeon to manipulate the touchscreen during the procedure. For optimal bone removal, we recommend assembling the CORI handpiece with a 5-mm spherical burr and speed control guard, as per the surgeon's preferences. Avoid wrapping the ankle with thick drapes during patient setup since it can make it harder to detect malleolar reference points for registration. Using a leg positioner, elevate the femur to 45° and flex the knee to 90° **(Fig. 10.11)**.

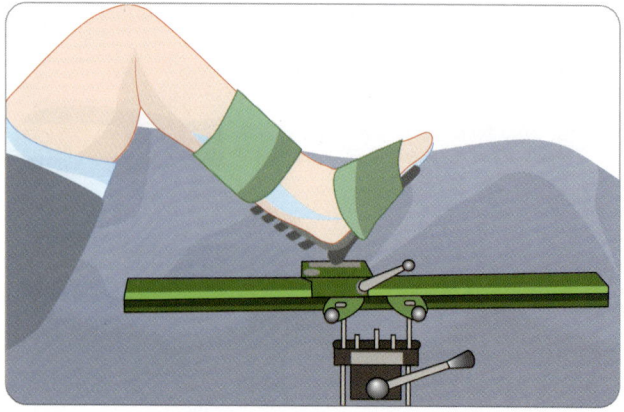

FIG. 10.10: Patient leg positioning.

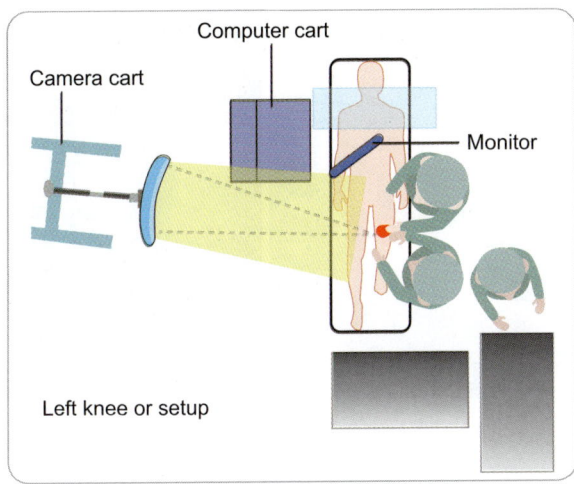

FIG. 10.11: Setup in operation room.

Making Incision/Arthrotomy

After subvastus/parapatellar incision depends on surgeon, check the joint and remove any visible spurs or osteophytes. To ensure accurate assessments of joint stability during virtual mapping and gap balancing, remove any peripheral osteophytes that may interfere with exposure. After resection and excision of osteophytes, the knee should be able to attain around 120° flexion.

Pin Placement with Drill Guide

In CORI-assisted surgery, achieving good results depends on securing the femoral and tibial tracking frames with a rigid, independent two-pin unicortical fixation.

For the tibial tracker, we place the first bone screw percutaneously about a handbreadth below the tibial tubercle on the medial side, drilling straight through the bone to engage the far cortex. After marking the site, we insert the second screw just below the first. We then attach the bone clamps and the tibial tracker, making sure the markers are clearly visible to the camera.

For the femoral tracker, we insert the first screw about a handbreadth above the patella. This can be done after the arthrotomy to avoid tethering the quadriceps or laterally before the arthrotomy, with the knee in deep flexion. Once the tracker is secured, we confirm that the markers stay in full view of the camera throughout the knee's range of motion (ROM) **(Figs. 10.12A and B)**.

We also place checkpoint pins in both the femur and tibia, keeping them away from resection areas, to monitor stability throughout the procedure.

Defining the Checkpoint (Figs. 10.13A and B)

- *Femur*: Medial side of condyle
- *Tibia*: Close to tibial tubercle and as lateral on the condyle

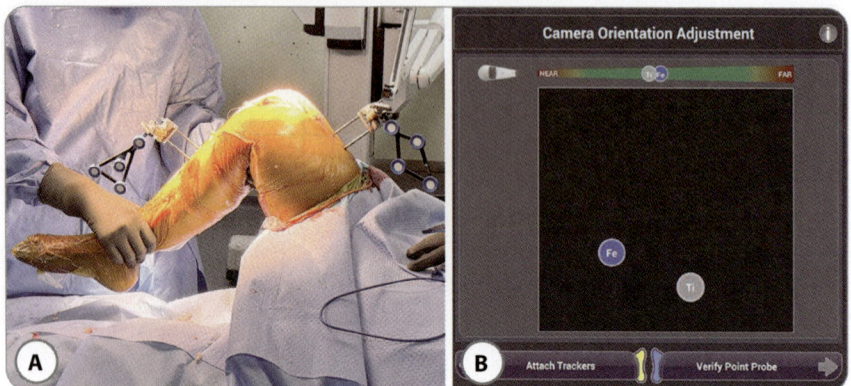

FIGS. 10.12A AND B: Trackers and camera orientation.

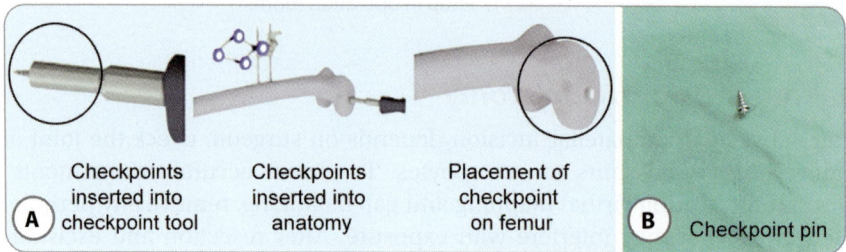

FIGS. 10.13A AND B: Checkpoint insertion.

Registration

CORI builds a virtual model of the patient's anatomy and kinematics using a CT-free registration procedure that is based on accepted image-free principles. To register the ankle center, the initial step in registration is to locate the most noticeable points on the medial and lateral malleoli using a point probe. Hip center computation, the following phase, uses circular hip movements to follow the femoral tracker array. Avoiding pelvic movement at this phase is crucial since it can lead to mistakes. The hip should be rotated gradually pressing and holding down the right foot pedal (hold), rotating the leg until all sectors are green. The femur should begin in about 20° of flexion (avoid hip flexion >45°) **(Fig. 10.14)**.

After that, fully extend the leg and press and hold the right foot pedal to determine the patient's varus/valgus alignment **(Fig. 10.15)**. The user can then record normal flexion motion using the preoperative knee motion collection interface. To achieve maximum flexion, move the leg through a normal (unstressed) ROM, collecting all conceivable sectors between at least 20° and 50° **(Fig. 10.16)**. Next, provide the collateral ligaments continuous varus and valgus stress while gathering data during flexion. The amount of laxity that should be incorporated into the corresponding medial and lateral gaps for appropriate joint balancing will be determined using this data.

CHAPTER 10: CORI Robotic System

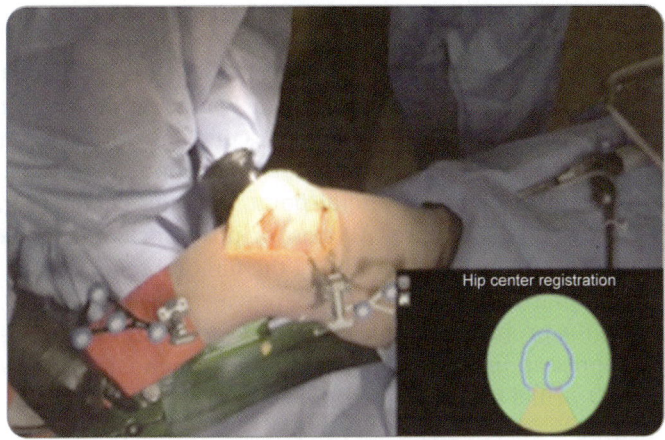

FIG. 10.14: Hip center registration.

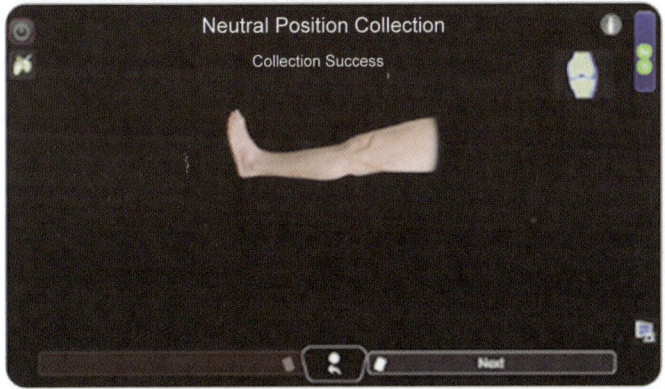

FIG. 10.15: Point collection with limb starting in neutral position.

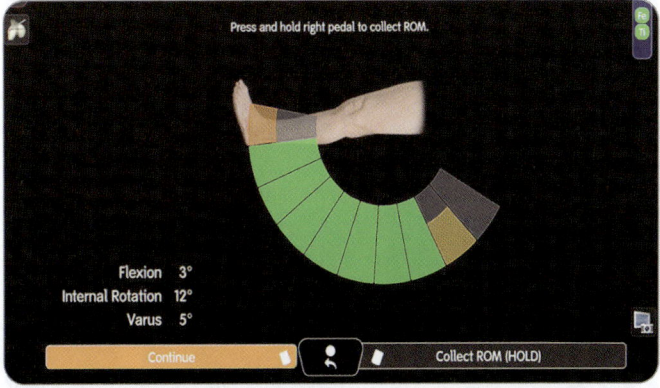

FIG. 10.16: Collect range of motion (ROM) from neutral to flexion of limb.

Performing Free Collection (Femur)

CORI Surgical Systems free collection stage allows you to characterize and understand the bony anatomy of the patient. Four landmark points need to be gathered in order to record the femoral condylar surfaces. Capture the knee utilizing the point probe, the anterior notch point, the most posterior medial point, the most posterior lateral point, and the center **(Fig. 10.17A)**. The transepicondylar axis, femoral AP axis, or posterior condylar axis are the three alternatives available for determining the femoral reference for rotational alignment, depending on the surgeon's preference.

At this point, the probe is "painted" over the whole femoral surface while the foot pedal is depressed in order to perform femoral condylar surface mapping **(Fig. 10.17B)**. 3D virtual model created.

Performing Free Collection (Tibia)

In the tibia while performing free collection the goal is to collect enough surface points on the tibial plateau. The knee center, medial plateau, and lateral plateau points are the three tibial landmarks that need to be collected **(Fig. 10.18A and B)**. The tibial rotational axis can then be defined using the four possibilities

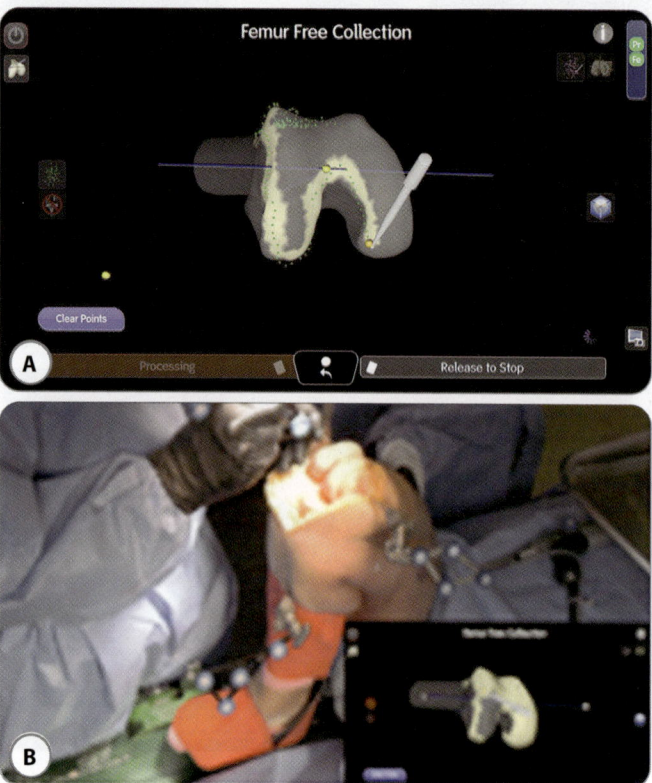

FIGS. 10.17A AND B: Femur free collection with 3D model.

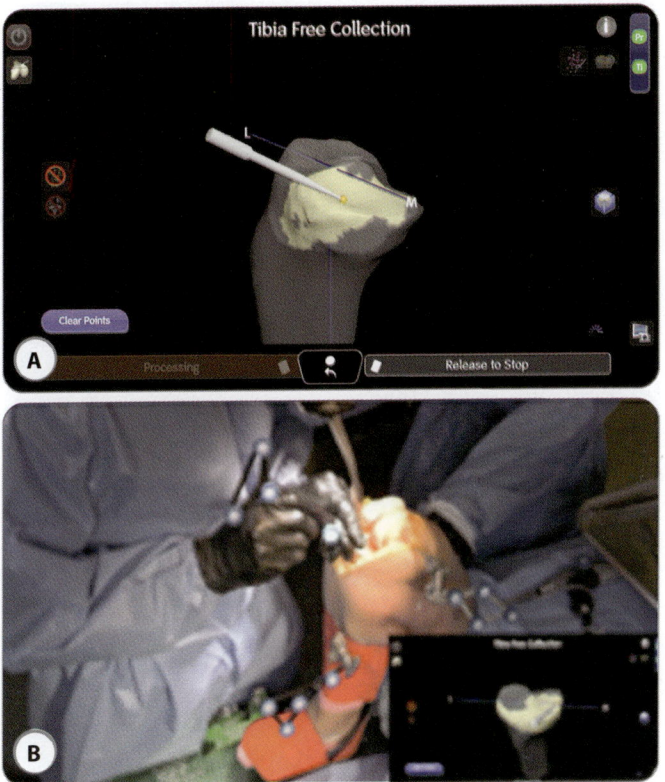

FIGS. 10.18A AND B: Tibia free collection with 3D model.

listed during the preceding surgical preference selection—the medial third of the tibial tubercle collection, the tibia anteroposterior (AP) axis, the medial lateral axis, and the transfer femoral mechanical axis. The previously gathered tibial mechanical and rotational axes can be visualized through the last registration step, tibial condyle surface mapping. Additionally, the user should digitize the tibial condylar surfaces by holding down the foot pedal while "painting" the point probe over the surface to create the virtual model.

Collecting Rotational Axis (Figs. 10.19A and B)

- The screen shows the previously defined M-L axis, and CORIO surgical system interprets the position of the point probe to create a virtual AP/ML axis live model.
- Reference for implant placement
- Surgeon-controlled femoral rotation preference

Implant Planning (Figs. 10.20A to C)

Initial sizing and placement, gap balancing, and cut guide placement are the three main steps in the CORI implant planning process. In order to prevent notching

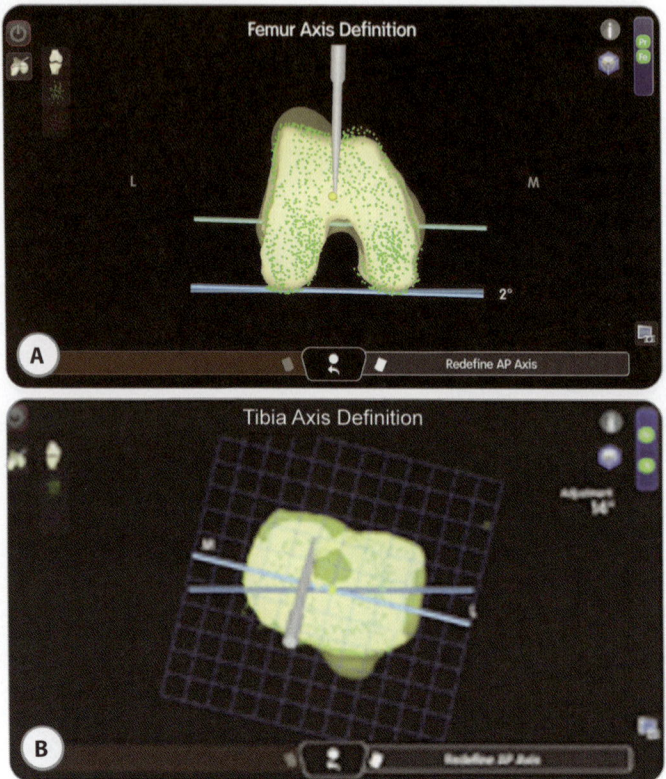

FIGS. 10.19A AND B: Defining rotational femur and tibia axis.

and ensure appropriate anterior transition and posterior covering, surgeons use cross-sectional and sagittal images to verify size and fit for the femoral component. Without compromising the anterior fit, the technology permits downsizing to adjust posterior gaps. The size, posterior slope, rotation, and resection depth of the tibial component are all adjusted once initial placement is determined by landmark data. For the best fit, thicker polyethylene inserts can alternatively be chosen.

Using virtual views, surgeons evaluate and modify virtual soft tissue tension over the whole ROM during the gap balancing stage. Achieving balanced extension and flexion gaps without medial or lateral overlap is the aim. Updated laxity data can be used to mimic virtual soft tissue releases and to modify the rotation and position of the implant. Throughout motion, the final implant placement is adjusted to maintain a constant 2–3-mm joint gap above the zero line.

Measuring ligament tension over the knee's ROM is part of the joint laxity assessment process. Digital tensioner **(Fig. 10.21)** is the first solution connected with a robotic system to quantify joint laxity prior to making any bony resections. Varus and valgus stress tests are given during full extension (−10° to +10°) to assess medial and lateral compartment tightness. The results are shown on a graph to help guide any necessary ligament releases. In order to measure joint

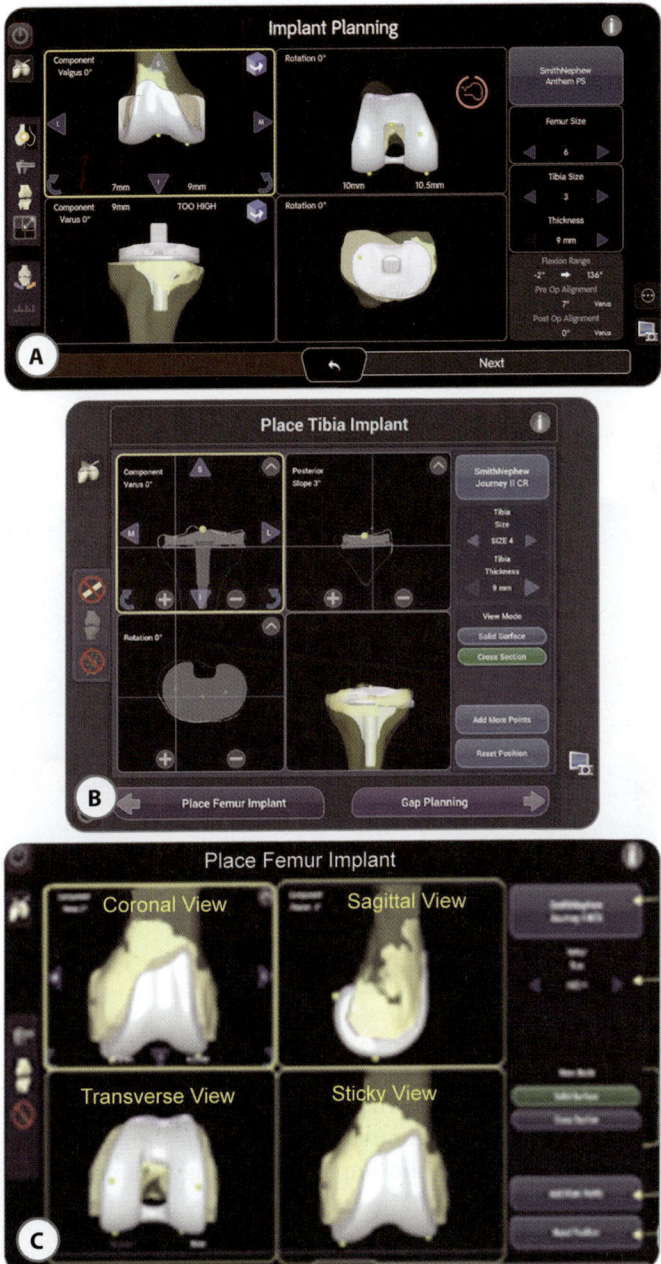

FIGS. 10.20A TO C: (A) Overall implant position on 3D model for femur and tibia; (B) tibial implant positioning; (C) Femur implant fit in all three view.

laxity in flexion, the knee is then flexed to 90° (80°–100° range), and comparable load is applied, frequently with the aid of instruments such as a digital tensioner, Z-retractor, or laminar spreader.

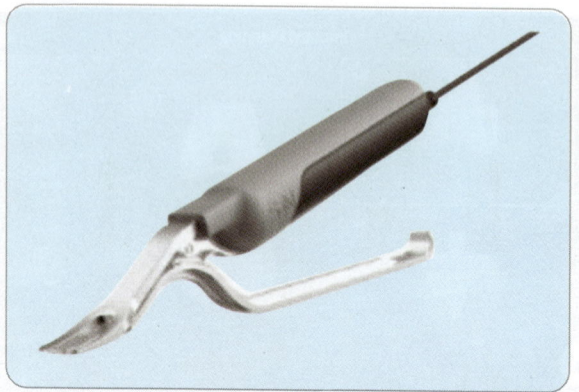

FIG. 10.21: Digital tensiometer.

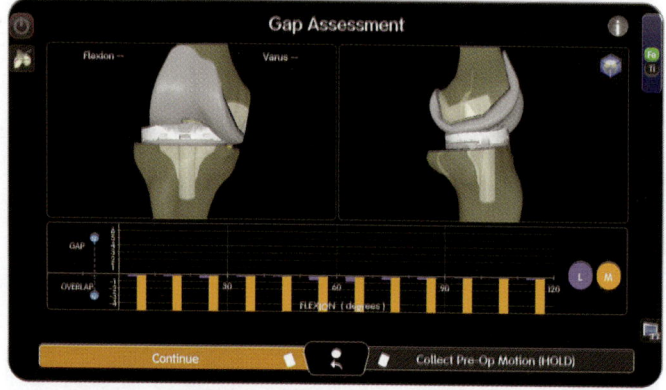

FIG. 10.22: GAP assessment.

Gap Planning (Fig. 10.22)
- For the medial compartment, the system turns orange, and for the lateral compartment, it turns purple. The medial compartment and lateral compartment gaps are plotted throughout the flexion range.
- The graph is translated to the implant planning screen to assist with gap balancing throughout the ROM.
- X axis—ROM in flexion
- Y axis—gap/overlap

Implant Planning with Gaps (Fig. 10.23)
- Continuous gap depicts the joint space and ligament laxity throughout the collected ROM.
- Confirm implant resection is appropriate avoiding notching and attention to the tibial slope.

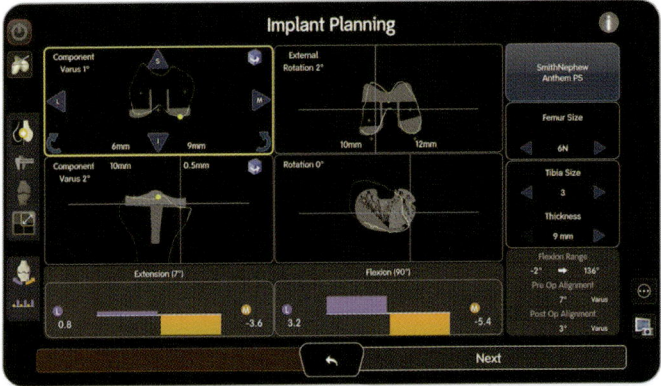

FIG. 10.23: Implant planning with gaps.

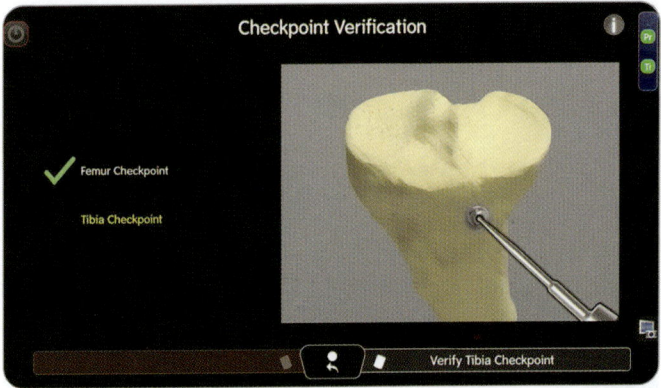

FIG. 10.24: Checkpoint verification.

Checkpoint Verification (Fig. 10.24)

The tick signals successful point collection.

Bone Cutting

Bone preparation for TKA utilizing the CORI system is usually done with a hybrid technique that combines saws and burrs. The default for TKA is Bur All. In accordance with the implant plan, the robotic handpiece positions cutting guides by creating exact lug slots. Accurate resection with a manual saw is made possible by the stabilizing block and pins that secure the distal femoral cut guide. Before finishing the femoral cuts, holes are drilled for the implant and a 5-in-1 cutting guide is positioned and verified with a plate probe **(Fig. 10.25)**.

Using the virtual plan as a guide, the robotic tool makes four lug slots for tibial resection. Two methods for performing bone removal on the tibia **(Fig. 10.26)** are Bur all and Twin Peg guide. The tibial cutting guide is then precisely positioned and fastened with pins. Soft tissue shields are utilized to prevent harm to the surrounding ligaments and tissues during the sawing resection of the tibia.

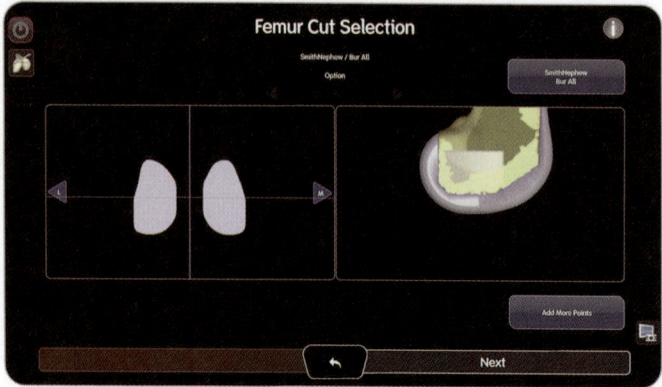

FIG. 10.25: Femur cut guide selection.

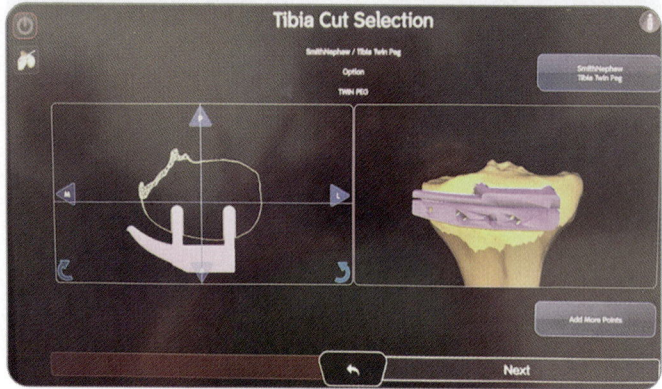

FIG. 10.26: Tibia cut guide selection.

Bone Removal (Figs. 10.27A and B)

Bur All method eliminates the need for the AP 5 in 1 (JOURNEY II), 4 IN 1 (LEGION/GENESIS II) **(Fig. 10.28)**, or Twin Peg cut guides **(Fig. 10.29 and Table 10.2)**.

Cut verification with help of tool will show how much accuracy achieved between planned cuts **(Figs. 10.30A and B)**.

TRIALING

While the femoral and tibial tracking arrays are placed, trial components are added in order to use clinical and virtual evaluation to evaluate knee motion, limb alignment, and varus/valgus balance along the whole flexion arc. Measurable information on medial and lateral laxity is available on the postoperative stressed gap assessment screen. Before finishing the last surface preparation for the manual implantation of the definitive components, additional bone or soft tissue adjustments can be done in light of these findings.

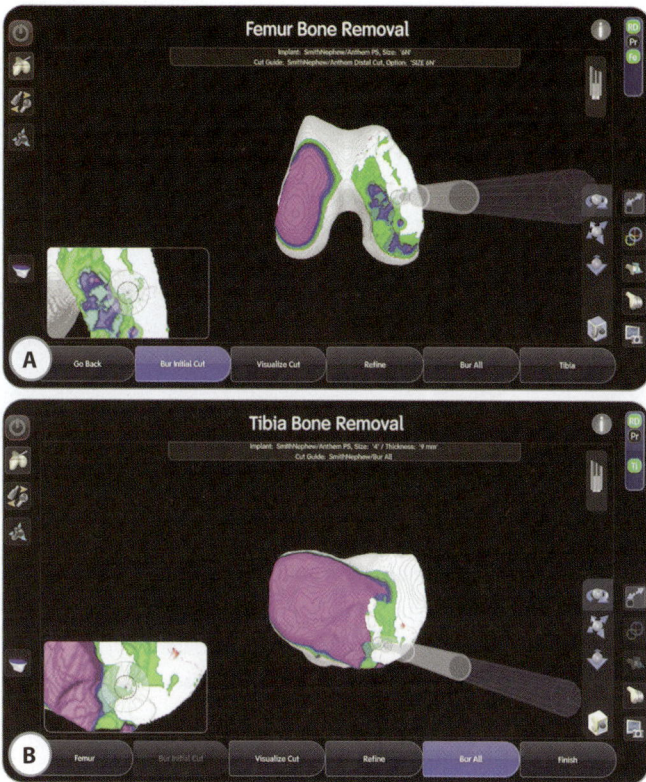

FIGS. 10.27A AND B: Femur bone removal and tibia bone removal.

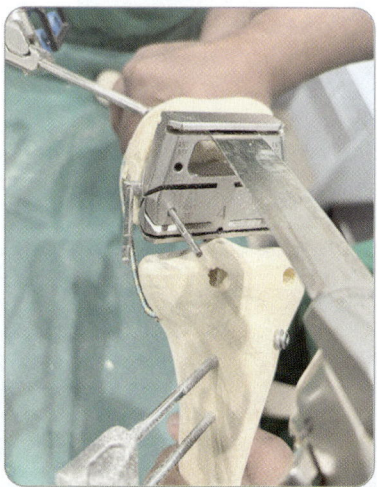

FIG. 10.28: Distal resection with anteroposterior cut guide (femur).

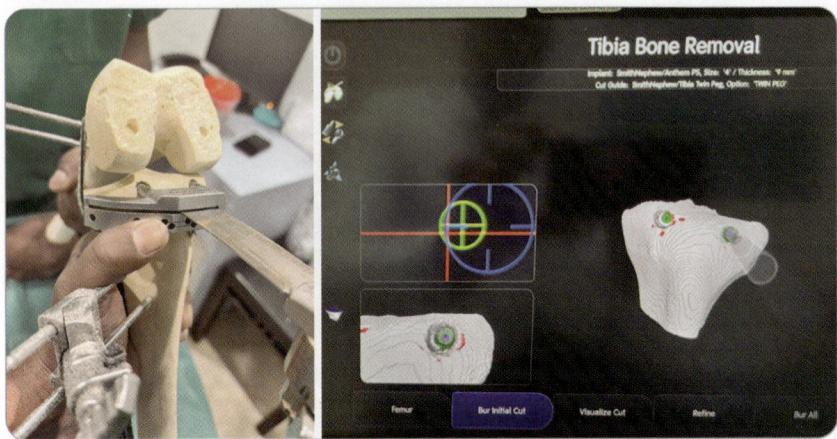

FIG. 10.29: Bone removal with twin peg cut guide (tibia).

TABLE 10.2: Color Guide to the Twin Peg Cut.	
Color	**Appropriate depth of bone to remove**
Magenta	>3 mm from target surface
Blue	Approximately 2 mm from target surface
Green	Approximately 1 mm from target surface
White	Approximate target surface
Red	Below target surface or more

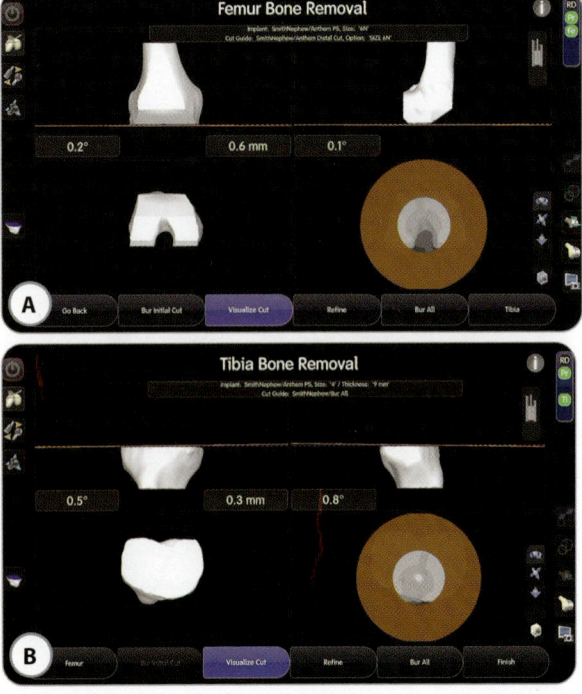

FIGS. 10.30A AND B: Visualizing bone removal (femur and tibia).

COLLECTING THE POSTOPERATIVE BASELINE

- Goal—collect postoperative baseline ROM **(Fig. 10.31)**
- CORI Surgical System uses the information collected to evaluate the knees postoperative ROM and gap assessment.

ASSESSING POSTOPERATIVE STRESSED GAP (FIG. 10.32)

Achieved varus/valgus is displayed, and the current line plot on the graph displays the stressed ROM from the gap planning stage.

Implant Trialing (Fig. 10.33)

Objective of this stage is to provide the surgeon with information pertaining to the TKA case.

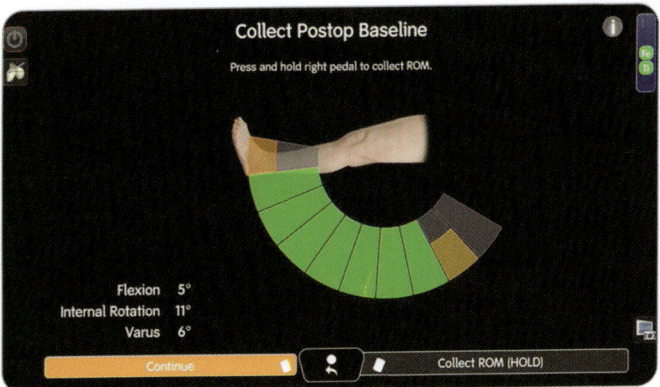

FIG. 10.31: Postoperative collection ROM.

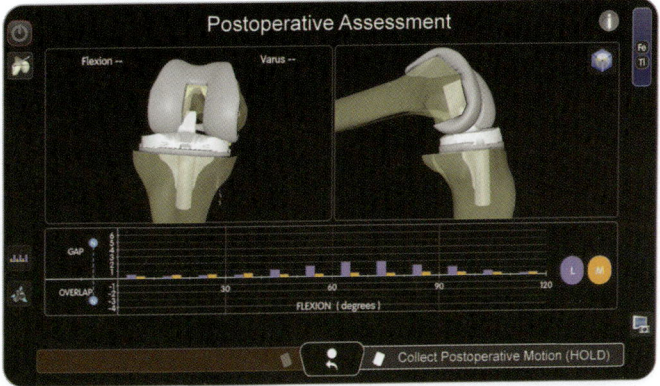

FIG. 10.32: Postoperative gap assessment with stressed ROM.

Inference

Advantages

- Compact design with 10-second calibration, fast process, 29% faster, 2X cutting volume, and 2x longer "throw" for easier posterior resection, boot up time 30 seconds
- Image-free real-time mapping and planning
- CT-free navigation spares patient exposure to extra radiation, saves patient and surgeon's time prior to procedure
- It saves the healthcare system incremental cost of CT
- Handheld robotics—reliable and consistent robotic-assisted bone preparation with handheld instrumentation
- Multiple supported implants, which have a good registry track record
- Proprietary STRIDE Knee system is optimized for robotic assistance
- Surgeon-controlled system
- Multimodality in bone preparation, Burr All, cut (saw capture) guide method, and Burr + Saw
- Options of changing the plan multiple times without having to go to the software. It can change the balance, alignment by taking a step back to the planning screen
- Real intelligence factors in the ligament laxity which is prerecorded before the cuts

Disadvantages

- High-speed burr can generate a lot of heat while cutting sclerotic bone on medial tibial plateau, hence irrigation is provided along with a suction tip to offset this disadvantage
- Bone debris aerosol is generated
- The handheld device is back heavy with a smaller grip ergonomically leading to fatigue of the smaller joints of the hand while operating and cutting through tough bone

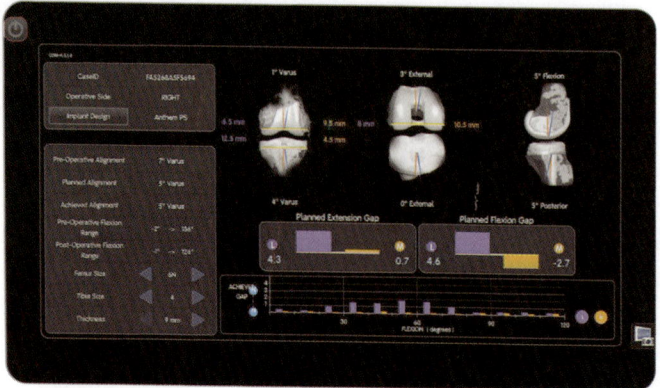

FIG. 10.33: Final gap with trial implant.

- The option for the saw capture requires a minimum bone cut of about 6 mm and can't be used in knees where the cut is going to be very conservative

TIPS AND TRICKS FOR SURGICAL PLANNING WITH THE CORI

After having morphed or drawn a picture of the patients knee with the anatomical landmarks the system creates a model with the osteophytes and gives the information of the axes along with the ligament laxity and overlap or tightness graph at the bottom of the screen.

The system also lets the surgeon plot a freehand points or landmarks called "special points".

One can make a smart use of the special points to doublecheck or crosscheck the computer-generated landmarks versus the anatomical land marks that the surgeon would have used in the conventional knee arthroplasty techniques.

There is a very easy interplay of the component positioning and sizing that can be done to effectively show the effect of the alignment and the sizing and positioning of the components on the ligament laxity and tightness in flexion and extension.

This happens in real-time enabling the surgeon to play with different alignment strategies and component positioning for the different deformities and the bone loss that the patient has.

These adjustments can be made either after an extensive release of the soft tissues and excision of the osteophytes as is done by many surgeons or can be done after.

We tend to do a moderate amount of release as a part of the exposure removal of the osteophytes and assess the balance as we would do it in a conventional technique. Then arrange or play with the femoral or tibial component positioning, alignment, and sizing to get a good balance.

It is our experience that a medial tightness of about 2–4 mm is easily tackled by the bony cuts and a slight recessing of the tight ligaments. The planning is done with a CR knee in mind.

ROSA Robotic System

Gaurav Kanade, Sanjay Dhar, Syed Mussadique Ali

■ INTRODUCTION

Total knee replacement (TKR) has seen significant advancements with the advent of robotic-assisted surgery, enhancing precision and consistency. The ROSA® (Robotic Surgical Assistant) Knee System, developed by Zimmer Biomet, stands out as a pioneering nonimage-based robotic platform, eliminating the need for preoperative CT or MRI scans. This system relies on intraoperative anatomical mapping and kinematic data to assist surgeons in achieving optimal implant positioning and alignment. Traditional TKR techniques, including conventional jig-based and early robotic-assisted methods, often depend on preoperative imaging for surgical planning. In contrast, ROSA® offers real-time data and adaptability during surgery, reducing preoperative costs, eliminating radiation exposure, and improving workflow efficiency. This chapter delves into the surgical workflow, accuracy, benefits over traditional techniques, and clinical outcomes of ROSA nonimage-based robotic TKR, highlighting its role in enhancing surgical precision and patient outcomes.

Robotic-assisted knee replacement has revolutionized joint arthroplasty by improving accuracy, efficiency, and patient outcomes. The *ROSA Knee System* (ROSA®) **(Fig. 11.1)** is a state-of-the-art robotic platform designed to enhance precision in TKR. This system integrates advanced *robotic arm technology, optical tracking, and planning software* to optimize intraoperative execution.

■ PRINCIPLES OF NONIMAGE-BASED NAVIGATION

Traditional robotic-assisted TKR often requires preoperative imaging, such as CT or MRI scans, to create a 3D model of the patient's anatomy for surgical planning. However, *ROSA's nonimage-based system eliminates this step*, relying instead on intraoperative data acquisition and real-time kinematic analysis.

The ROSA® Knee System operates on the principle of inverse kinematic alignment (iKA), which aims to maintain the native tibial joint line obliquity and balance the flexion and extension gaps by adjusting femoral resections. This

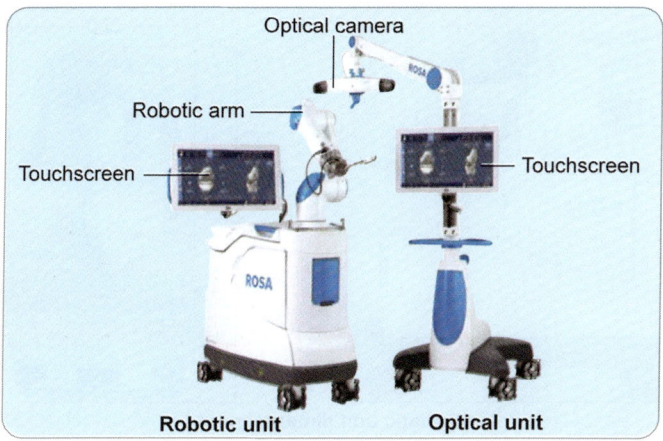

FIG. 11.1: ROSA Knee System.

approach contrasts with traditional mechanical alignment (MA), which corrects every leg to a hip-knee-ankle (HKA) angle of 180°. The iKA strategy reduces the need for ligamentous or capsular releases, thereby minimizing the risk of knee instability and improving biomechanics. The ROSA Knee System primarily operates on the principle of *iKA* but can also support *MA and restricted kinematic alignment (rKA)* based on surgeon preference.

Specifications

Physical Characteristics
- *Size and shape*: Compact, mobile system with an ergonomic design
- *Weight*: Robotic unit weight: Approximately 320 kg (705 lb); optical unit weight: Approximately 140 kg (309 lb)
- Footprint size **(Figs. 11.2A to D)**
- *Minimum area required*: 400 meters for safe and optimal working radius
- *Design language*: Modular structure for easy maneuverability and positioning

Robotic Arm Specifications
- *Axes and accuracy*: ROSA knee is equipped with a Stäubli six-axis robotic arm and has 6° of freedom.
- Working radius **(Figs. 11.3A and B)**
- Optical tracking system

The optical unit is composed of **(Fig. 11.4)**:
- Optical camera
- Camera positioning arm
- Touchscreen

Camera
- *Type*: Infrared-based optical tracking
- *Vision angle*: Wide angle

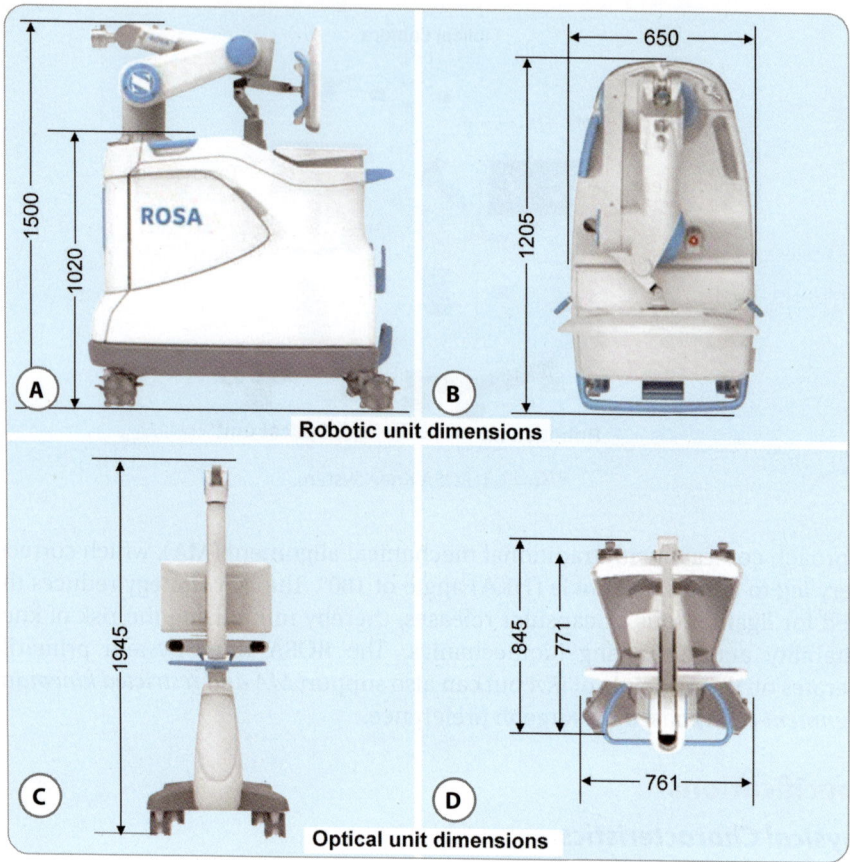

FIGS. 11.2A TO D: ROSA Knee System dimensions.

Optical Trackers
- *Type*: Active/passive tracking
- *Shape*: Flat
- *Lifespan*: Use unblemished trackers; each is single use.

Note: Although not recommended by the company, trackers can be reused if cleaned and sterilized properly for at least 20–25 cases.

Plane (Arrays/Markers)
- *Formation*: Multiplane tracking arrays
- *Margin of error*: Very less for real-time positional tracking

Interactive Device
- *Monitor specifications*: High-definition touch-screen interface for real-time feedback

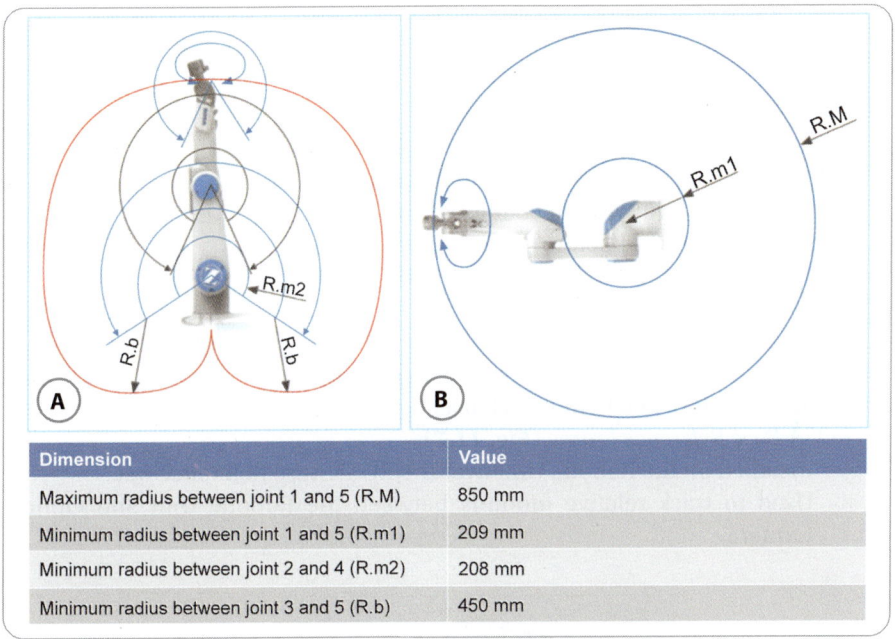

Dimension	Value
Maximum radius between joint 1 and 5 (R.M)	850 mm
Minimum radius between joint 1 and 5 (R.m1)	209 mm
Minimum radius between joint 2 and 4 (R.m2)	208 mm
Minimum radius between joint 3 and 5 (R.b)	450 mm

FIGS. 11.3A AND B: Working radius of ROSA Knee System.

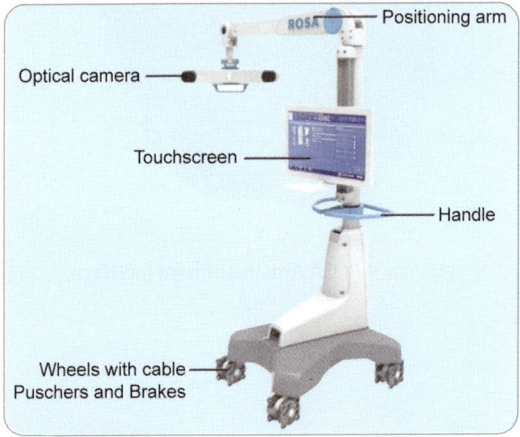

FIG. 11.4: Components of optical tracking system.

Cutting system: High-precision oscillating saw for bone resection:
- *Standard surgical tool*: It uses a regular high-precision oscillating saw, not attached to the robot.
- *Manual operation*: Surgeon manually operates the saw for bone resection.
- *Robotic guidance*: Robotic arm guides the saw to the precise location for cutting.
- *Precision*: Ensures accurate bone cuts, crucial for optimal implant placement.
- *Safety*: Controlled oscillation minimizes risk to surrounding tissues.

ROSA® Knee System Instrumentation and Assembly Overview

Instrumentation

- *ROSA Arm Instrument Interface (Fig. 11.5)*:
  - Attached to the robotic arm with three captive screws.
  - Maintains sterility when changing tools.
  - Must be sterilized before each use.
  - Use handles to hold during installation to preserve sterility.
- *ROSA Arm Reference Frame (Fig. 11.6)*:
  - Attached to the Robotic Arm interface with two captive screws.
  - Used for Robotic Unit registration before surgery.
  - Must be sterilized before each use.
- *ROSA Base Reference Frame (Fig. 11.7)*:
  - Installed on the Robotic Unit over the ROSA Base Reference Bar.
  - Used to track relative motions between the Robotic Unit and Optical Camera.

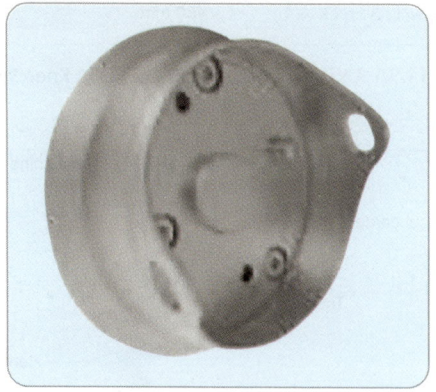

FIG. 11.5: ROSA Arm Instrument Interface.

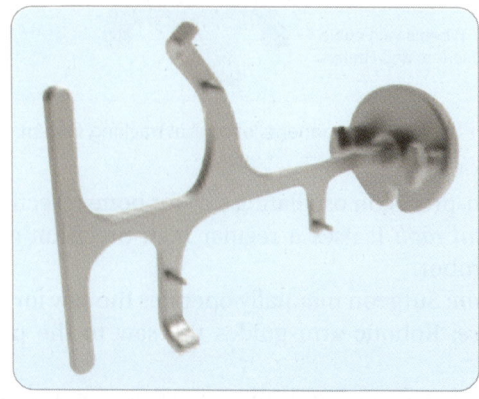

FIG. 11.6: Arm Reference Frame.

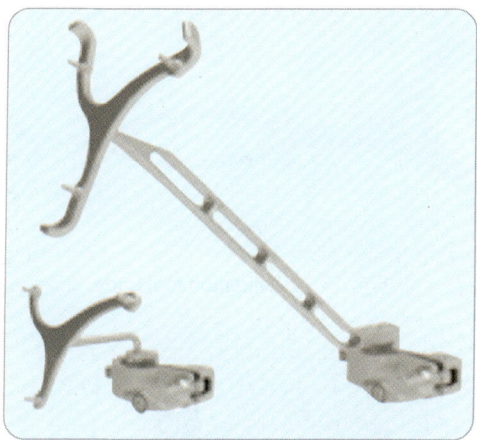

FIG. 11.7: Base Reference Frame.

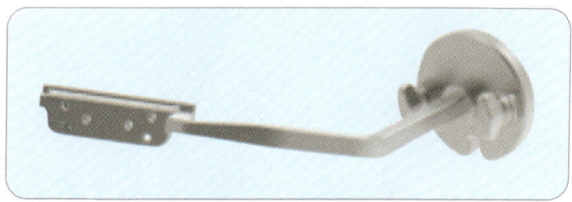

FIG. 11.8: Total knee arthroplasty cut guide.

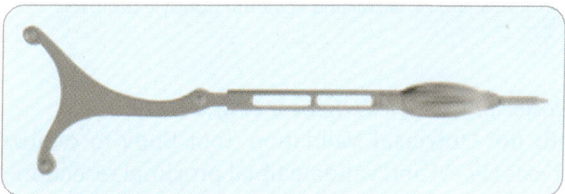

FIG. 11.9: Registration pointer.

- o Must be sterilized before each use.
- o If it moves during surgery, re-register the Robotic Arm.
- *ROSA TKA Cut Guide (Fig. 11.8)*:
  - o Attached to the ROSA Arm Instrument Interface with two captive screws
  - o Two versions (A and B) based on the surgeon's and Robotic Unit's position relative to the patient
- *ROSA registration pointer (Fig. 11.9)*:
  - o Used to digitize anatomical landmarks.
  - o Must be sterilized before each use.
  - o Avoid piercing cartilage with the tip.
- *Universal validation tool body (Fig. 11.10)*:
  - o Used to validate femoral distal resection.
  - o Must be sterilized before each use.

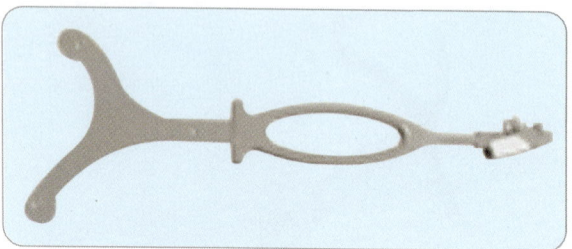

FIG. 11.10: Validation tool body.

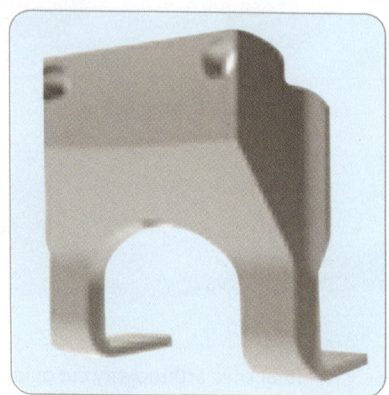

FIG. 11.11: Distal and Posterior Condyle Digitizer.

- *Distal and Posterior Condyles Digitizer (Fig. 11.11)*:
  - Used with the Universal Validation Tool Body to digitize the posterior condylar axis (PCA) and validate tibial proximal resection.
  - Must be sterilized before each use.
- *ROSA Knee Condyle Digitizer (Small/Medium/Large)*:
  - Used with the Universal Validation Tool Body to digitize the PCA.
  - Three sizes available; select based on patient anatomy and surgeon preference.
  - Must be sterilized before each use.
- *ROSA Knee Tibia Validation Tool (Fig. 11.12)*:
  - Used with the Universal Validation Tool Body to validate tibial resection.
  - Must be sterilized before each use.
- *Patient references*: Femoral reference frame *(Fig. 11.13)*: Fixed outside or inside the incision using percutaneous pins.
- *Tibial Reference Frame A/B (Figs. 11.14A and B)*: Fixed outside or inside the incision using percutaneous pins.
- Fixed using percutaneous pins into the medial surface of the tibial diaphysis.
- Must be sterilized before each use.
- Verify proper fixation of pins and references.

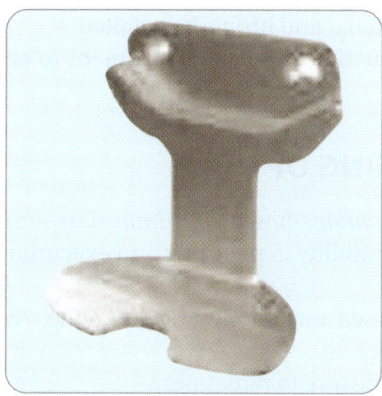

FIG. 11.12: Knee Tibia Validation Tool.

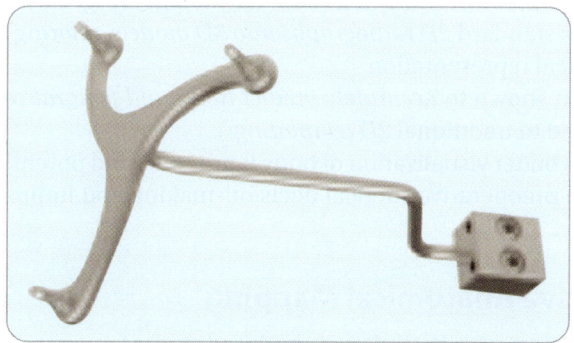

FIG. 11.13: Femoral reference frame.

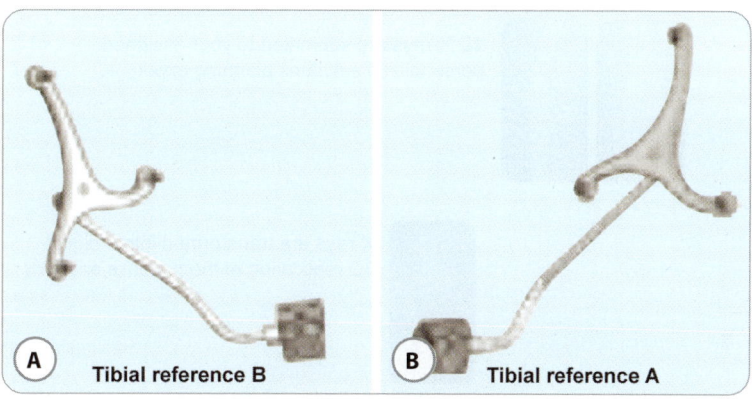

FIGS. 11.14A AND B: Tibial reference frames.

Summary

- All instruments must be sterilized before each use.
- Verify proper fixation of pins and references.
- Use handles to hold instruments during installation to preserve sterility.

- Ensure trackers are clean and properly installed.
- Follow specific instructions for each instrument to ensure accurate and safe use.

FLEXIBLE IMAGING OPTIONS

ROSA knee offers both *image-based and imageless options* based on surgeon preference, providing flexibility in planning and execution.
- *Imageless option*:
  - Eliminates the need for preoperative imaging, reducing overall surgical preparation time.
  - Limits patient exposure to radiation.
  - Addresses reimbursement concerns in certain healthcare systems.
  - Reduces scheduling constraints, allowing for streamlined case planning.
- *Image-based option (X-Atlas® 2D to 3D Technology)* **(Fig. 11.15)**:
  - Converts standard *2D radiographs into 3D models*, offering a more precise anatomical representation.
  - Has been shown to *accurately predict tibial and femoral component sizes* compared to traditional *2D templating*.
  - Provides better visualization of bony landmarks and potential deformities.
  - Helps in preoperative surgical decision-making and improves implant fit accuracy.

Intraoperative Anatomical Mapping

- The ROSA system uses *optical trackers* placed on the femur and tibia to register anatomical landmarks.

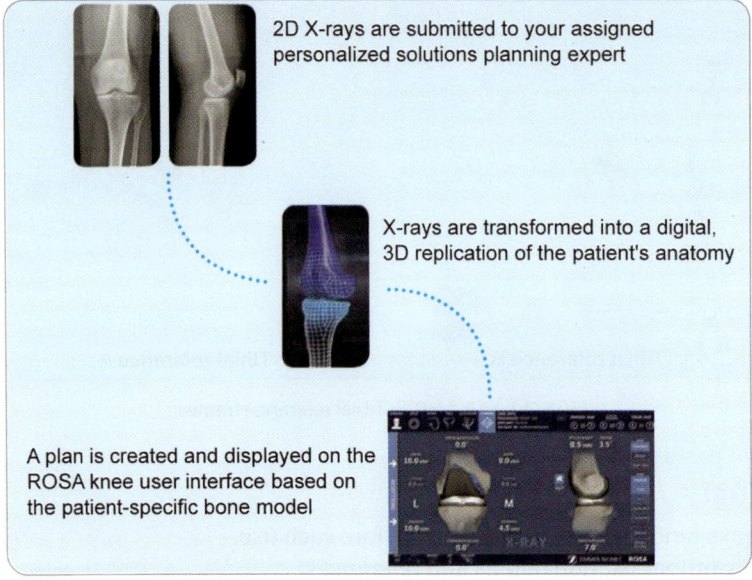

FIG. 11.15: Image-based Option (X-Atlas® 2D to 3D Technology).

- The surgeon manually identifies key reference points, such as the *hip center, femoral condyles, tibial plateau, and ankle center*, which are then digitized by the system.
- This data is used to create a *virtual model of the patient's knee*, guiding bone resections, and implant positioning.

Real-time Kinematic Assessment

- ROSA collects *dynamic motion data* by passively flexing and extending the knee intraoperatively.
- This allows the system to analyze *ligament balance, joint alignment, and soft tissue tension* in real time.
- Unlike static preoperative imaging, this dynamic assessment helps *optimize implant placement based on functional knee movement*, leading to better patient-specific results.

No Radiation or Preoperative Imaging

- Since no CT or MRI is required, *patients avoid radiation exposure and additional costs*.
- The system adapts intraoperatively, making it beneficial for cases with *severe deformities or altered bony anatomy*, where preoperative imaging may not be accurate.

The combination of *intraoperative anatomical registration and kinematic tracking* enables *precise and adaptive implant positioning*, improving surgical accuracy and patient outcomes.

Key Features

- *iKA*: This method focuses on maintaining the native joint line obliquity and balancing the knee joint through femoral resection adjustments.
- *No preoperative imaging*: Unlike other robotic systems, ROSA® does not require preoperative CT or MRI scans, reducing radiation exposure and simplifying the workflow.
- *Real-time adjustments*: The system provides real-time feedback and adjusts resections intraoperatively, enhancing precision and adaptability.

SURGICAL WORKFLOW OF ROSA NONIMAGE-BASED ROBOTIC TKR

The ROSA® Knee System integrates real-time data acquisition, robotic assistance, and surgeon-controlled execution to enhance precision in TKR. The surgical workflow consists of the following key steps.

Preoperative Setup (Figs. 11.16A and B)

Patient Positioning

The patient is placed in the standard supine position with the knee exposed for surgical access.

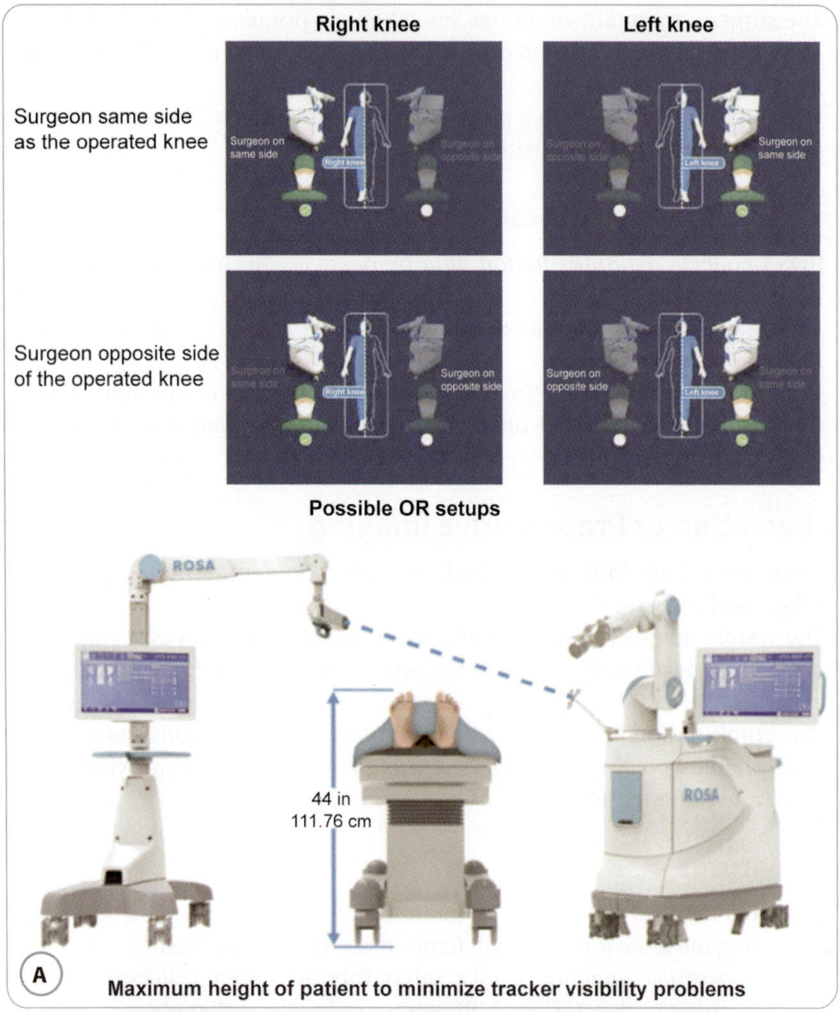

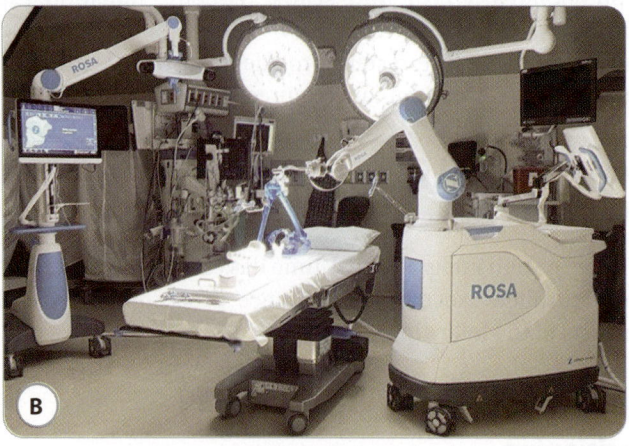

FIGS. 11.16A AND B: (A) Possible or setups and optimal patient positioning; (B) Ideal operation theatre setup for ROSA Knee System.

There are four possible OR setups:
1. Operating on a right knee, with the surgeon on the same side as the operated knee
2. Operating on a right knee, with the surgeon on the opposite side of the operated knee
3. Operating on a left knee, with the surgeon on the same side as the operated knee
4. Operating on a left knee, with the surgeon on the opposite side of the operated knee

Draping of robot (Fig. 11.17):
- *Sterile covering*: Ensure complete draping to maintain sterility.
- *Component protection*: Secure all robotic arms and sensors to prevent contamination.
- *Field accessibility*: Maintain clear access to the surgical site while preserving sterility.

Tracker Placement

Optical tracking arrays are securely fixed to the distal femur and proximal tibia to facilitate continuous real-time movement tracking.

Femoral reference placement outside the incision (Fig. 11.18):
- Place the knee in flexion to install the femoral reference.
- Use two fixed fluted pins 3.2 × 150 mm to install the patient femoral reference.
- Position the pins four fingers proximal to the knee incision to stay clear of the working area.
  - The pins can be inserted percutaneously through the vastus medialis in the femur.
  - The pins should be set near-bicortically in the bone to ensure maximum stability.
- Position the reference close to the skin (without compression or soft tissue impingement) and tighten the two screws to secure to the pins.

Femoral reference placement inside the incision:
- Bone reference installation **(Figs. 11.19A and B)**.
- Position the pins two fingers proximal to the proximal edge of the trochlea.

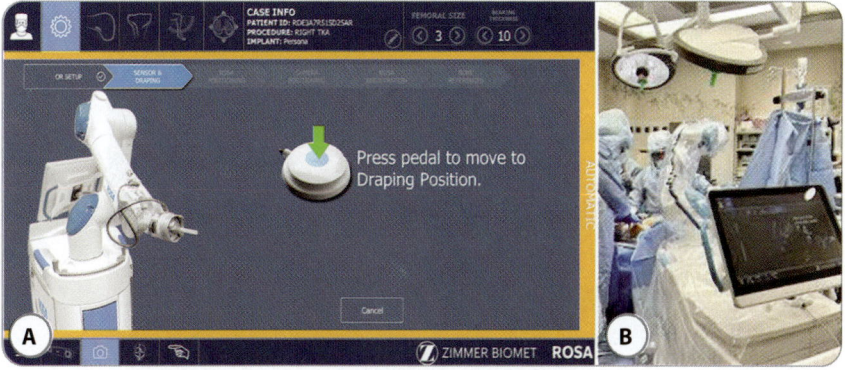

FIGS. 11.17A AND B: (A) Application to put rosa system in draping position; (B) ROSA draping completed.

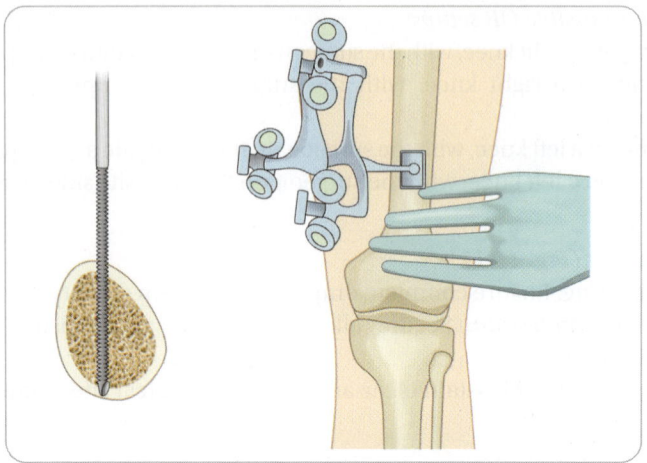

FIG. 11.18: External femoral reference placement.

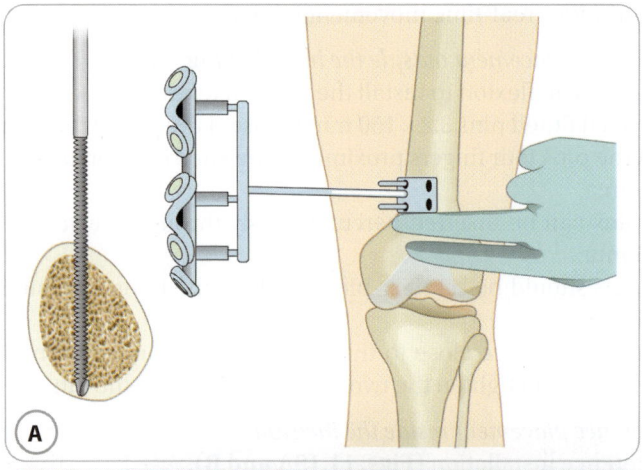

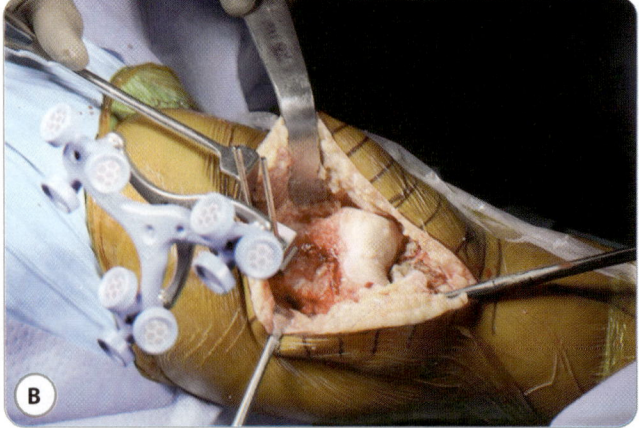

FIGS. 11.19A AND B: (A) Femoral reference placement inside the incision; (B) Clinical picture of femoral reference placement inside incision.

- Tilt the femoral reference toward the camera to avoid interference or contact between the femoral reference and the power tools, ROSA Cut Guide, implant, or bone pins and screws. The pins should be set bicortically in the bone to ensure maximum stability.
- Position the reference close to the bone/skin (without compression or soft tissue impingement) and tighten the two screws to secure to the pins.
- *Tibial reference placement outside the incision* (**Figs. 11.20A and B**):
  - Position the pins four fingers distal to the knee incision to stay clear of the working area.
  - The pins can be inserted percutaneously perpendicular to the medial surface of the tibial diaphysis.
  - The pins should be set near-bicortically in the bone to ensure maximum stability.
  - Position the reference close to the skin (without compression or soft tissue impingement) and tighten the two screws to secure to the pins.
- Tibial Reference Placement Inside the Incision (**Figs. 11.21**)
  - *Position the pins*:
    - Three fingers distal to the joint line—(1) on the anterior cortex, (2) distal, and (3) medial to the articular surface and the anticipated position of the ROSA Cut Guide.

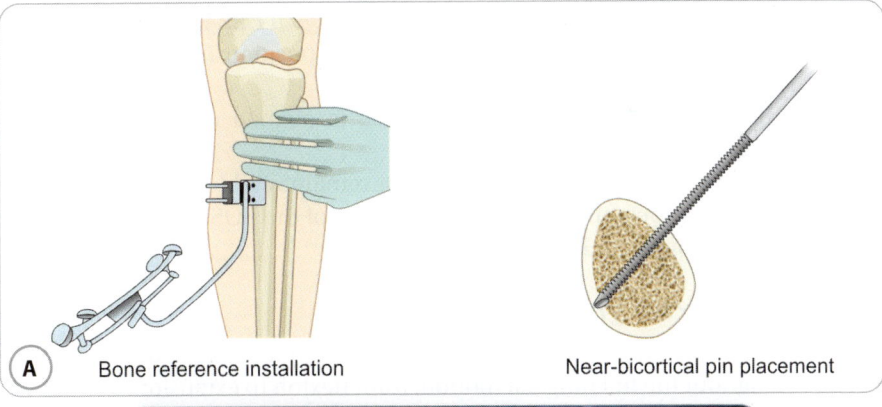

A Bone reference installation   Near-bicortical pin placement

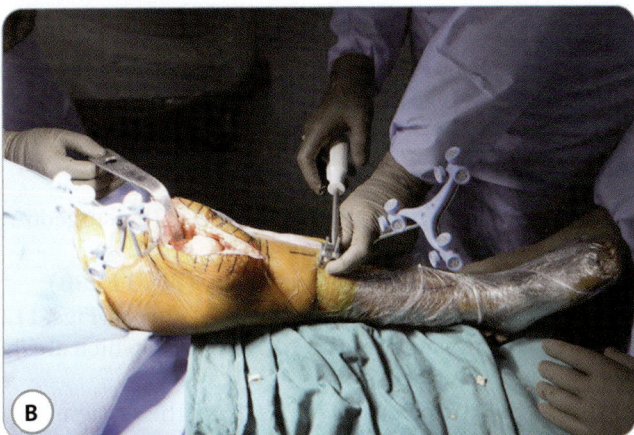

B

FIGS. 11.20A AND B: (A) Tibial reference placement outside the incision; (B) Clinical picture of tibial reference placement outside the incision.

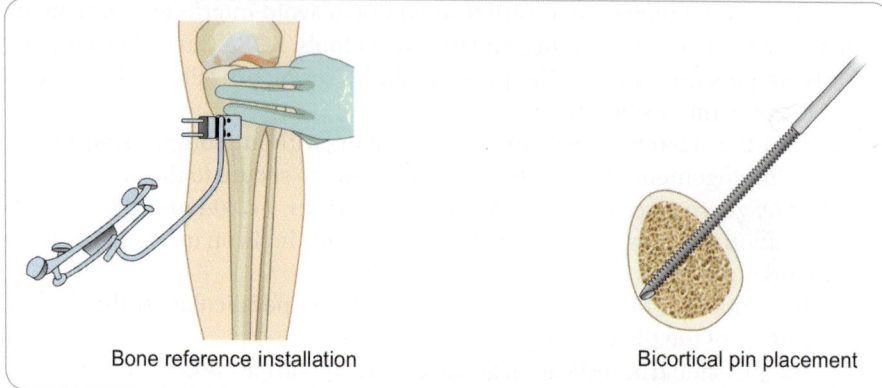

FIG. 11.21: Tibial reference placement inside the incision.

- The pins should be set bicortically in the bone to ensure maximum stability.
    - Position the reference close to the bone/skin (without compression or soft tissue impingement) and tighten the two screws to secure to the pins.
- *Moving ROSA and aligning the arm reference* **(Figs. 11.22A and B)**:
    - Initial positioning: Move the ROSA robot into position and align the robotic arm reference correctly before proceeding.
    - Verification: Ensure the arm reference is aligned accurately to avoid intraoperative deviations.
    - Stability check: Confirm that the robot remains stable and does not shift during the procedure. The final positioning of the ROSA system should be ideal as depicted in **Figures 11.23A and B**.

Navigation Tracker Visibility (Fig. 11.24)

Always check the position of the navigation tracker once installed. It should be visible throughout the full range of motion, from flexion to extension.

ROSA Registration **(Fig. 11.25)**:
- *System initialization*: Ensure all required components are properly connected and functional before proceeding with registration.

Intraoperative Registration

- *Anatomical landmark digitization* **(Fig. 11.26A)**: The surgeon registers key anatomical points, including:
    - Hip center (by passive movement of the leg) **(Fig. 11.26B)**
    - Medial and lateral femoral condyles, anterior cortex **(Figs. 11.26C and F)**
    - Tibial plateau and malleoli **(Figs. 11.27A and B)**, which are then digitized by the system.
- *Dynamic kinematic assessment* **(Fig. 11.28)**: The system captures knee motion through passive flexion-extension to evaluate soft tissue balance and alignment.

CHAPTER 11: ROSA Robotic System

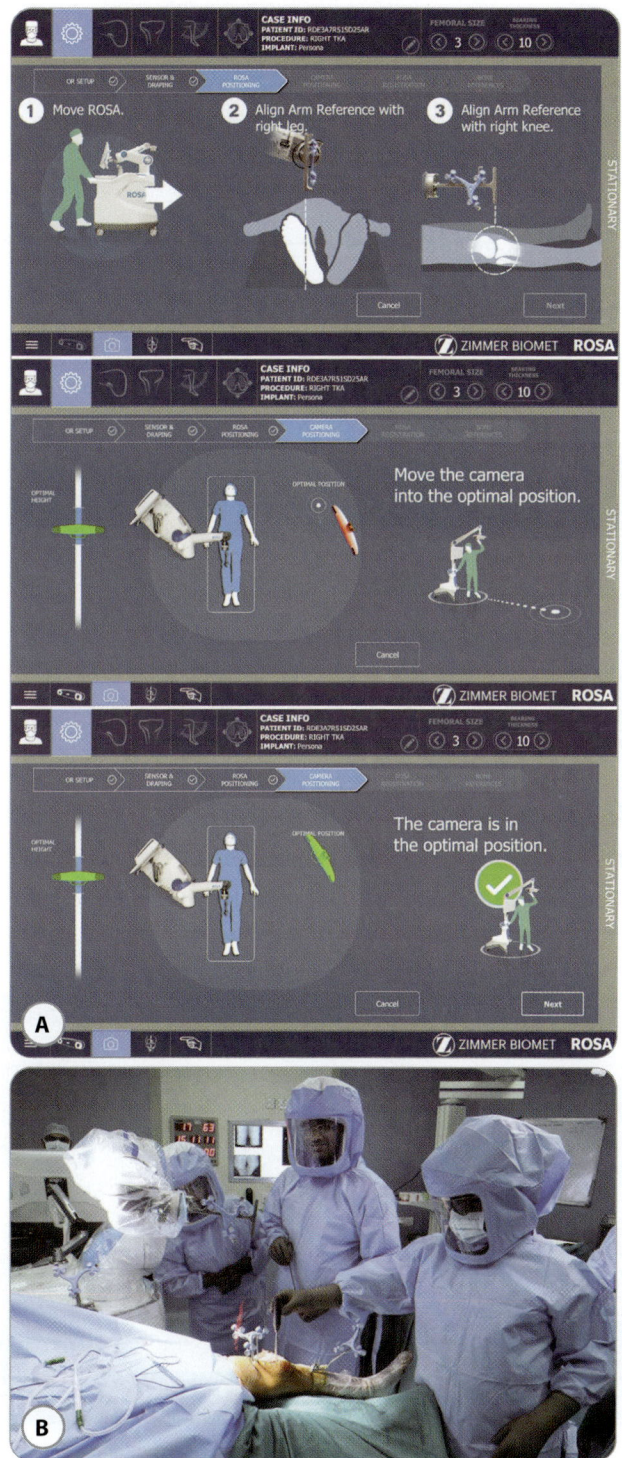

FIGS. 11.22A AND B: Moving ROSA and aligning the arm reference with optimal camera position; (B) Clinical picture.

CHAPTER 11: ROSA Robotic System

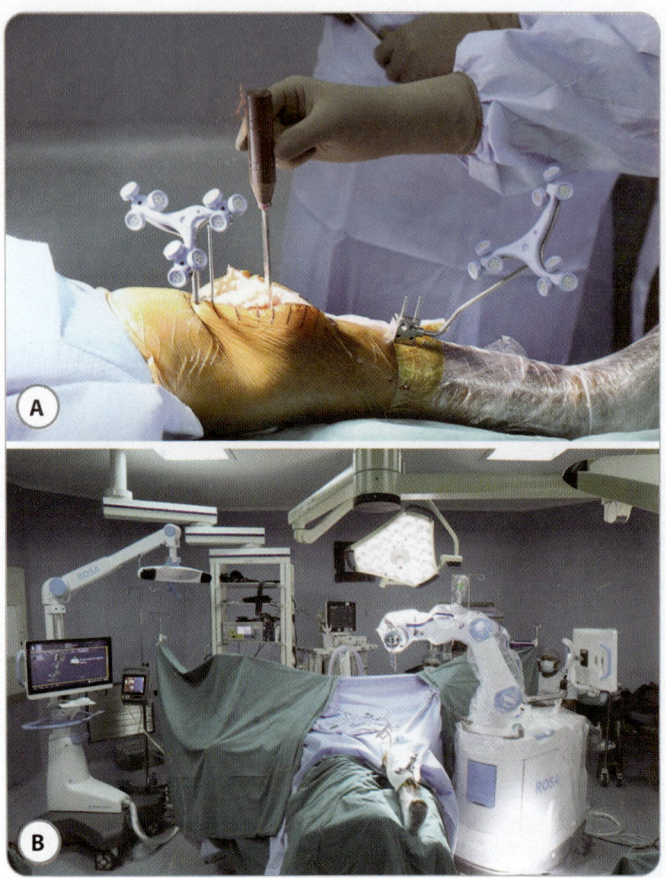

FIGS. 11.23A AND B: Final ROSA OT setup postdraping and optimal patient/camera positioning.

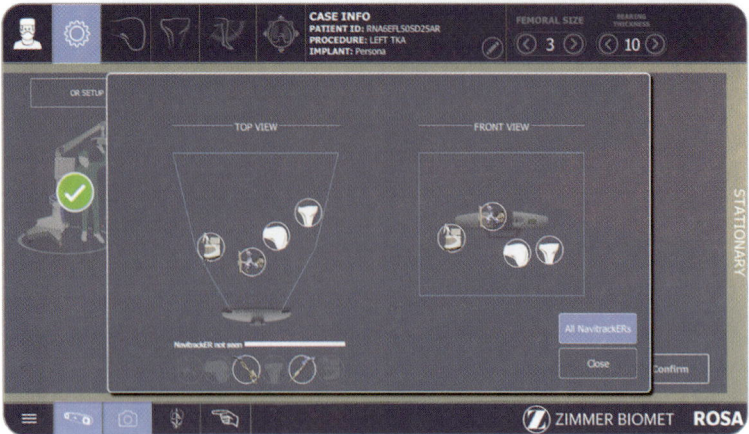

FIG. 11.24: Confirmation of navigation tracker visibility.

CHAPTER 11: ROSA Robotic System

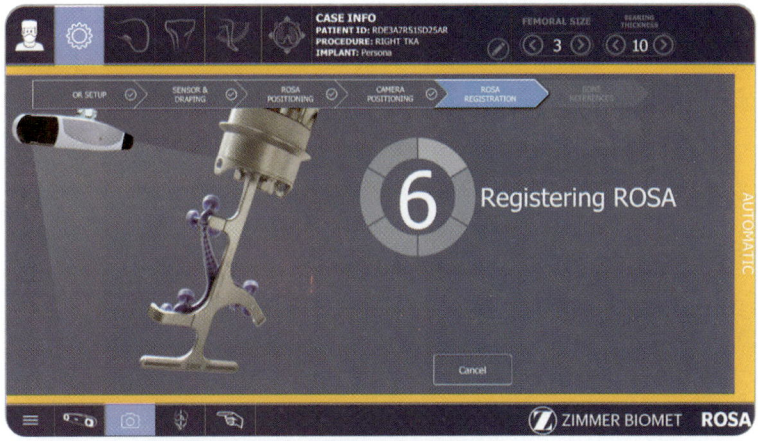

FIG. 11.25: ROSA registration.

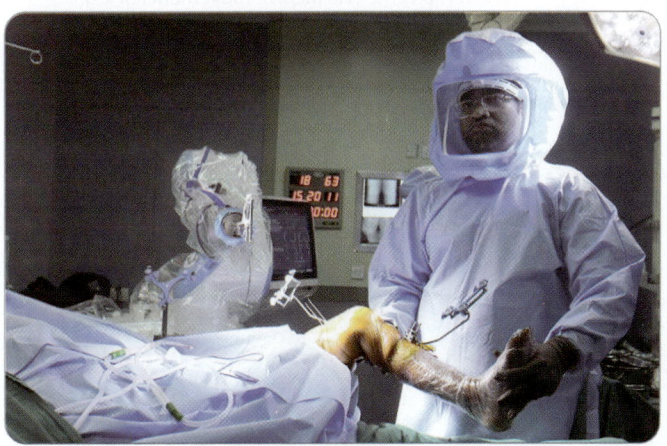

FIG. 11.26A: Anatomical landmark digitalization.

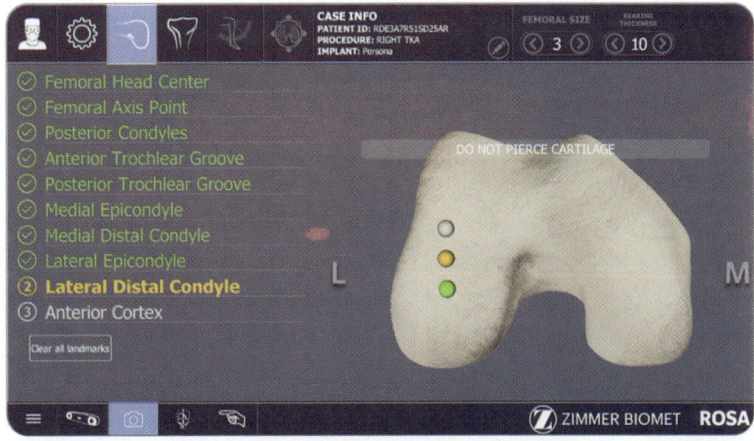

FIG. 11.26B: *Continued*

Continued

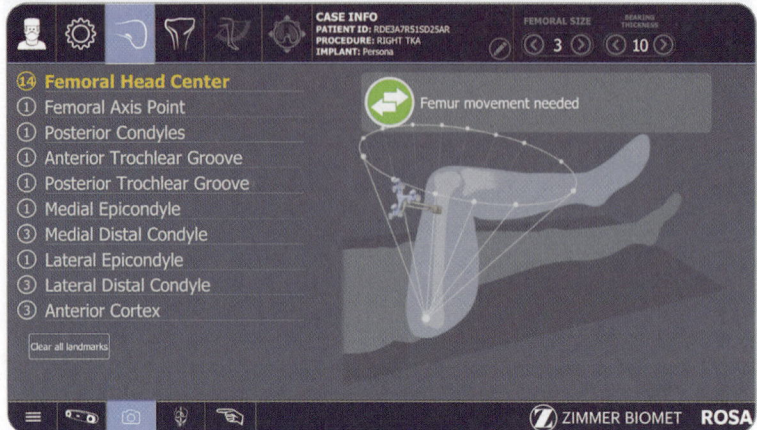

FIG. 11.26B: Hip center via passive movements of leg.

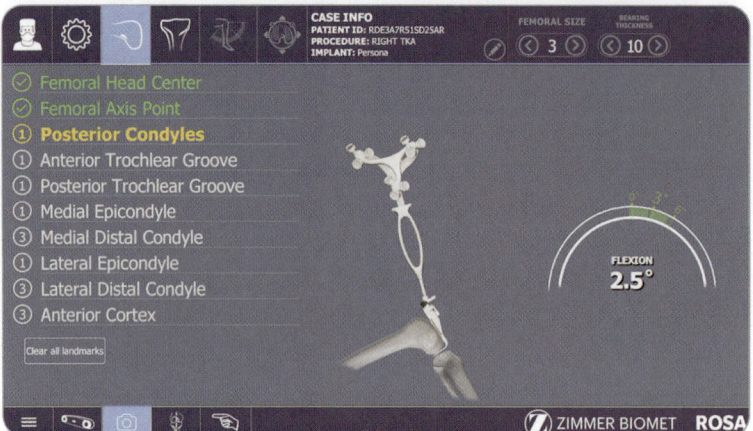

FIG. 11.26C: Anatomic landmark digitization of posterior condyles.

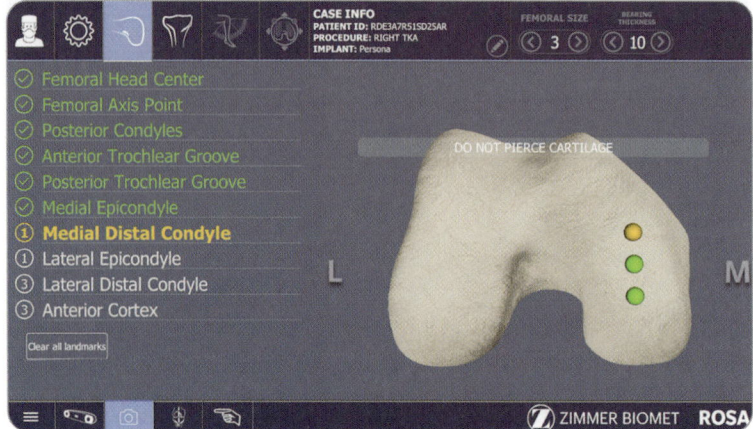

FIG. 11.26D: Anatomic landmark digitization of medial distal condyle.

CHAPTER 11: ROSA Robotic System

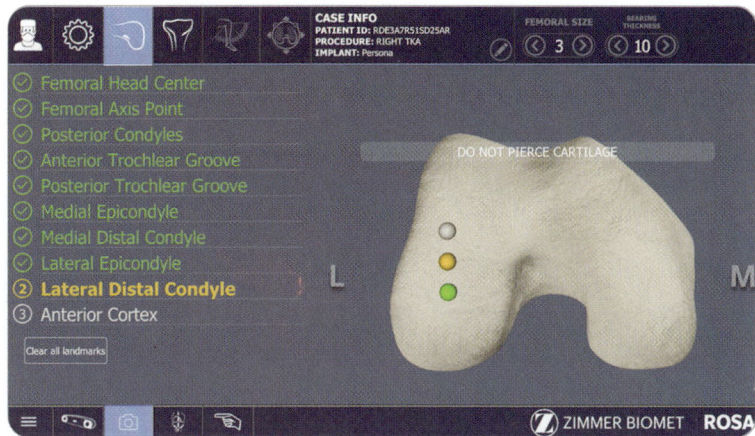

FIG. 11.26E: Anatomic landmark digitization of lateral distal condyle.

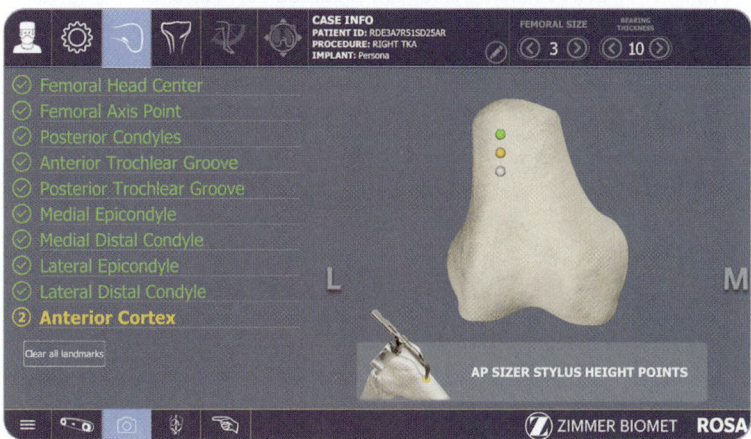

FIG. 11.26F: Anatomic landmark digitization of anterior cortex.

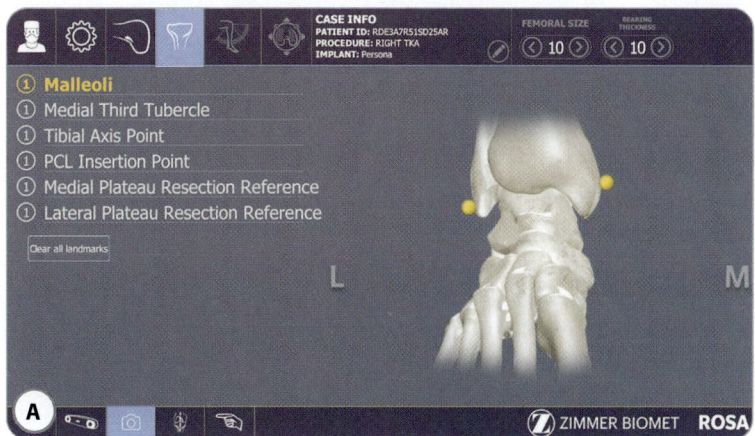

FIGS. 11.27A AND B: *Continued*

Continued

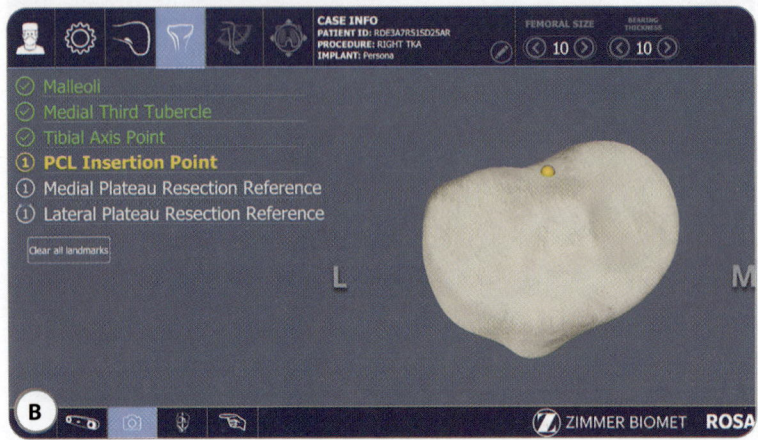

FIGS. 11.27A AND B: (A) Anatomic landmark digitization of malleoli of tibia; (B) Anatomic landmark digitization of posterior cruciate ligament (PCL) insertion point and tibial plateau.

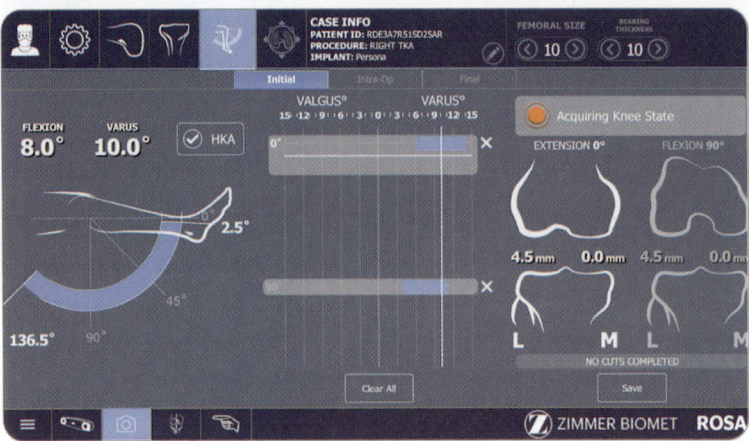

FIG. 11.28: Dynamic kinematic assessment.

Bone Resection Guidance (Fig. 11.29)

- *Virtual planning*: Based on intraoperative data, the system generates a patient-specific surgical plan.
- Bone resection planned by surgeon **(Fig. 11.30)**
- *Robotic-assisted bone cuts*: The surgeon executes femoral **(Figs. 11.31A to J)** and tibial **(Figs. 11.32A to C)** resections with robotic assistance, ensuring precision. ROSA provides real-time feedback on:
  - Varus/valgus alignment
  - Flexion/extension balance
  - Posterior condylar offset and tibial slope

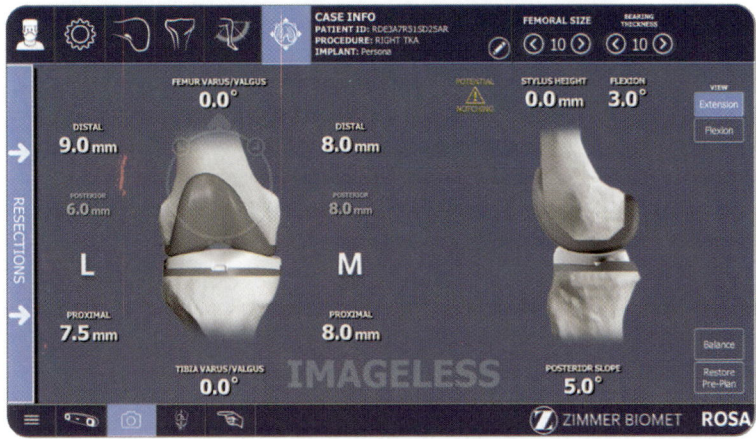

FIG. 11.29: Bone resection guidance.

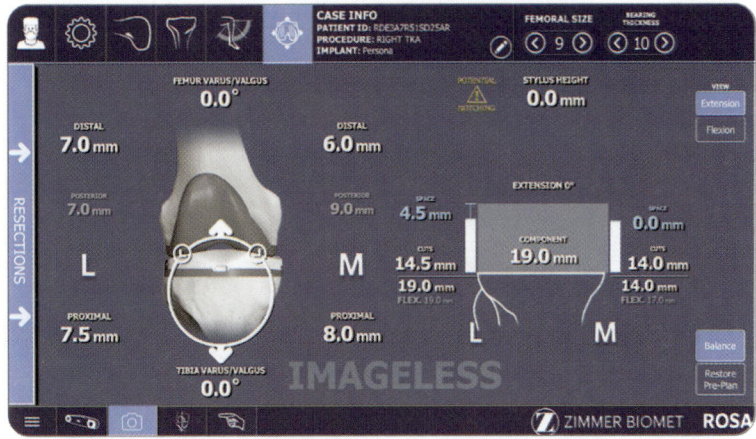

FIG. 11.30: Final bone resection planned by surgeon.

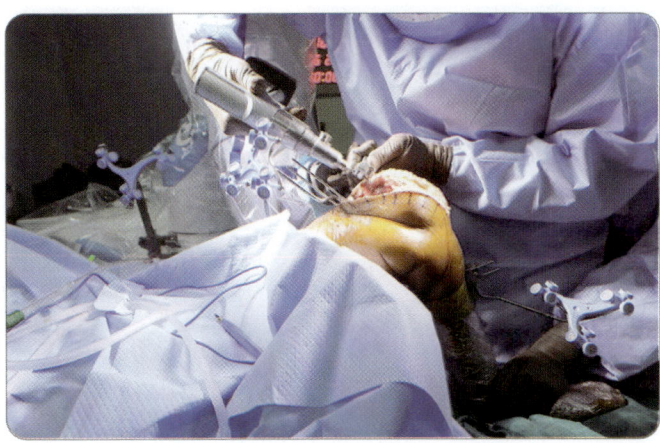

FIG. 11.31A (1): Robotic-assisted bone cuts (placement of distal femoral cutting jig).

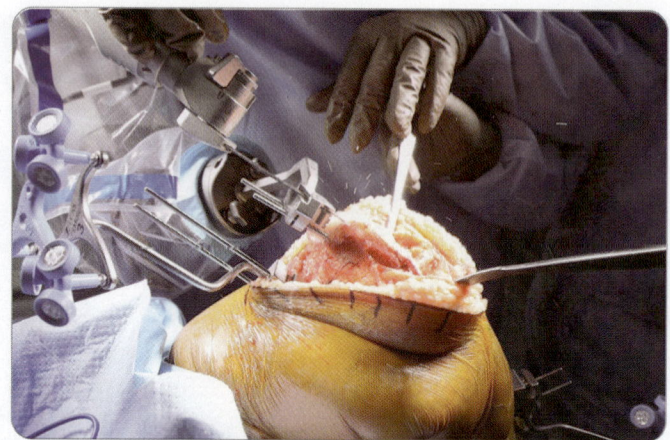

FIG. 11.31A (2): Femoral cuts taken with help of saw.

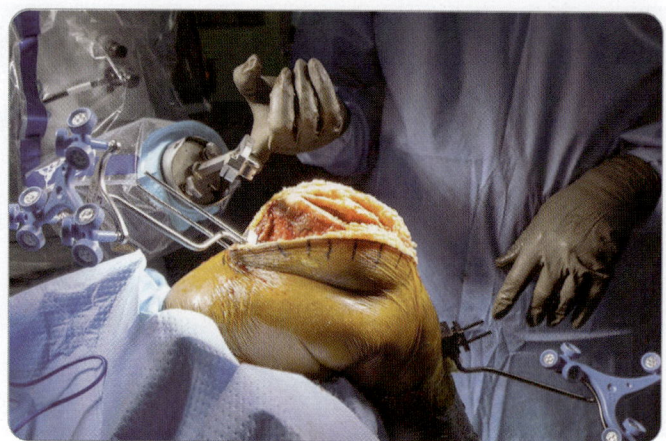

FIG 11.31B: Removing of the femoral cutting jig.

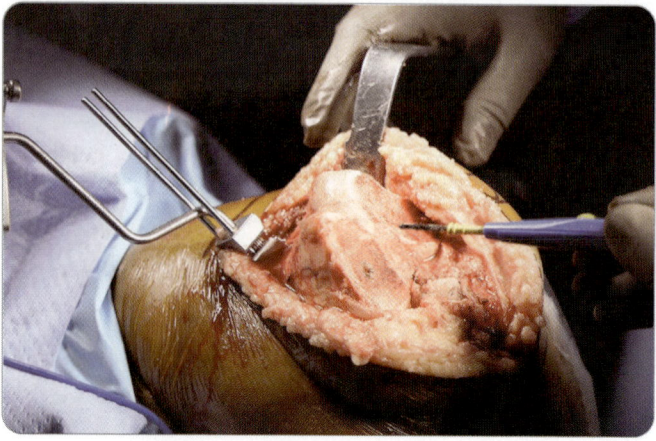

FIG. 11.31C: Final distal femoral bone cut.

CHAPTER 11: ROSA Robotic System 163

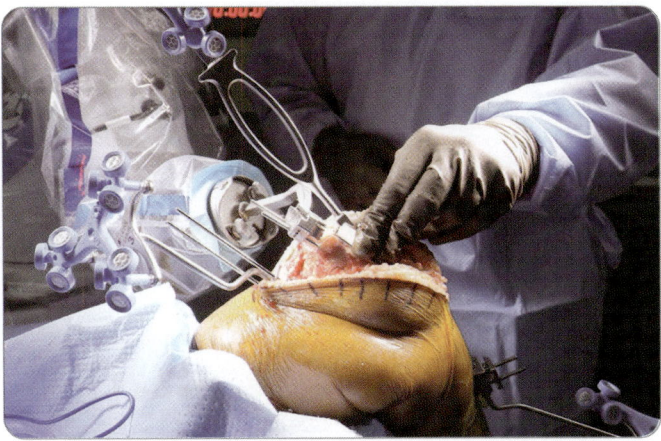

FIG. 11.31D: Confirming distal femoral cuts with validation tool.

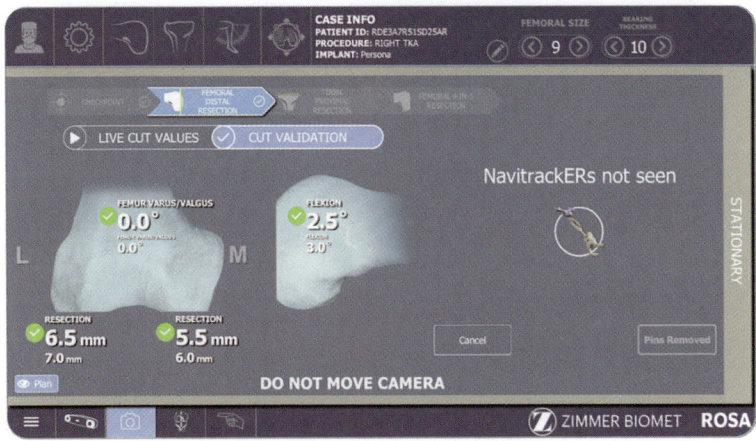

FIG. 11.31E: Confirmation of distal femoral cuts via ROSA system.

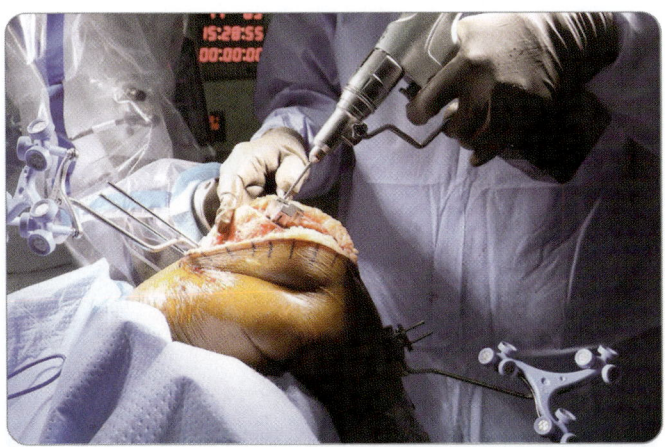

FIG. 11.31F: Robotic-guided pin-hole placement for 4-in-1 femoral cuts.

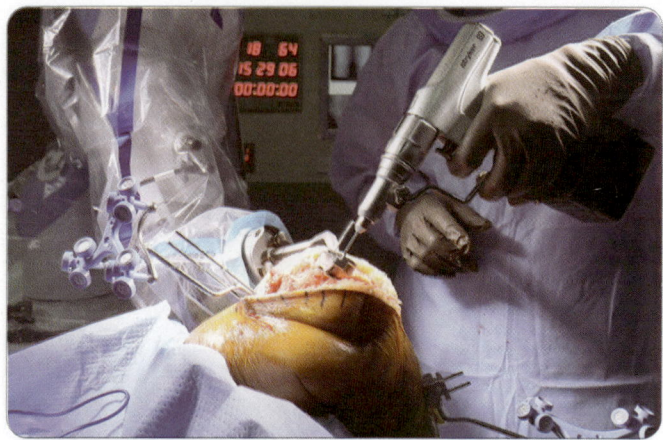

FIG. 11.31G: Robotic-guided pin-hole placement for 4-in-1 femoral cuts.

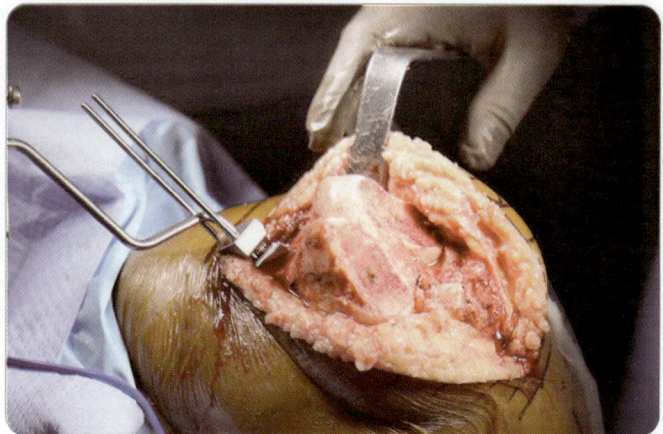

FIG. 11.31H: Robotic-guided pin-hole placement for 4-in-1 femoral cuts (completed).

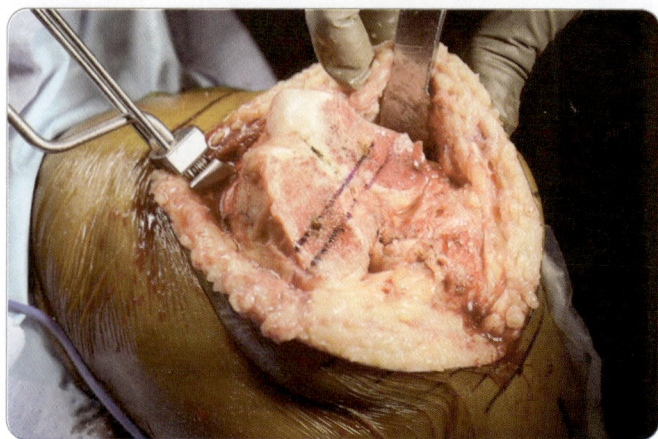

FIG. 11.31I (1): Rotation alignment checked: 4-in-1 cutting block pins versus transepicondylar axis.

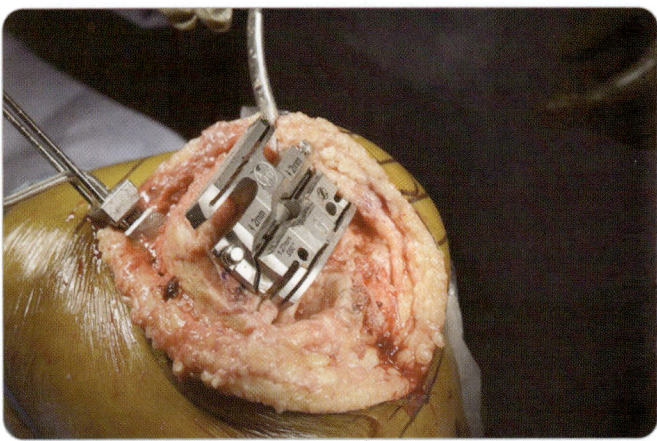

FIG. 11.31I (2): Placement of 4-in-1 cutting jig.

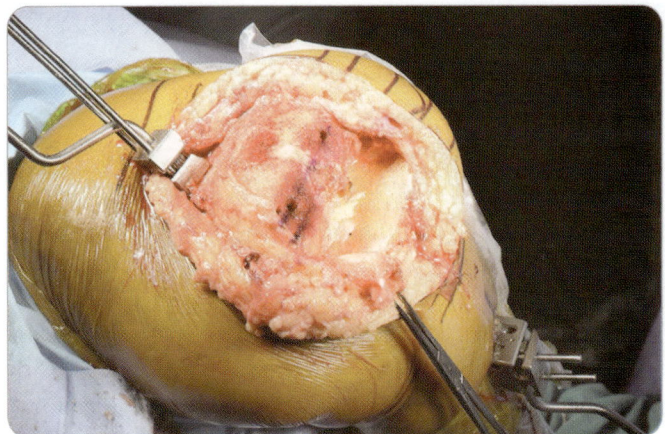

FIG. 11.31J: Clinical picture after completion of 4-in-1 cut.

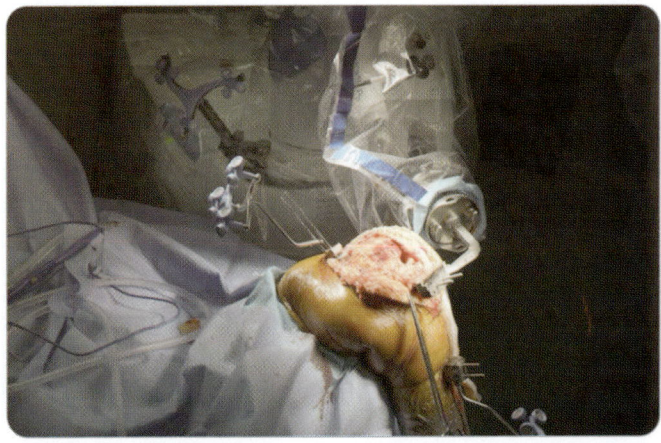

FIG. 11.32A: Robotic-assisted bone cuts (placement of proximal tibial cutting jig).

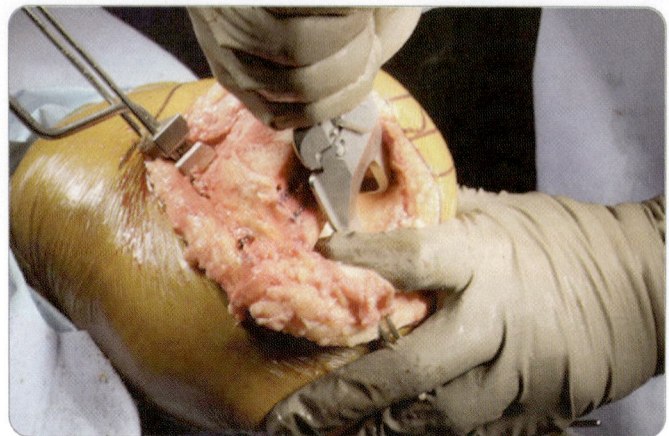

FIG. 11.32B: Confirming proximal tibial cut with validation tool.

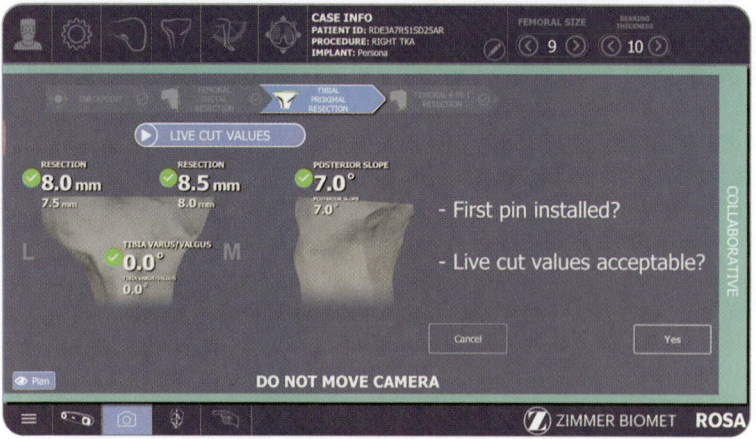

FIG. 11.32C: Confirmation of proximal tibial cuts via ROSA system.

Trialing and Soft Tissue Balancing

- *Trial implants* **(Fig. 11.33A)**: After bone preparation, trial implants are placed, and knee stability is reassessed.
- *Soft tissue balancing* **(Fig. 11.33A to C)**: The system provides feedback on gap balancing, ligament tension, and range of motion before final implantation.

Final Implant Placement (Fig. 11.34A to E) and Verification

- *Optimal alignment and balance*: Once optimal alignment and balance are achieved, the final prosthetic components are implanted.
- *Final kinematic check* **(Fig. 11.35)**: A final kinematic check ensures proper function before wound closure.

CHAPTER 11: ROSA Robotic System

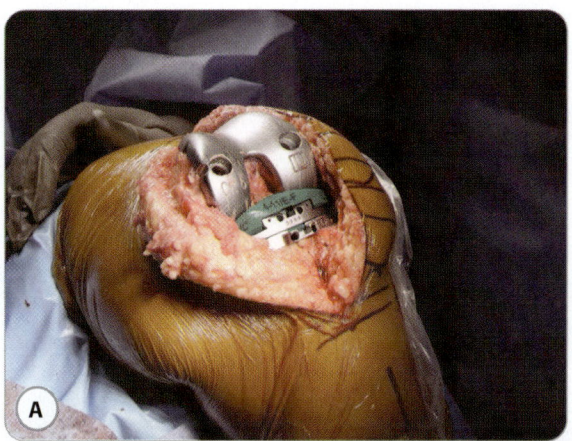

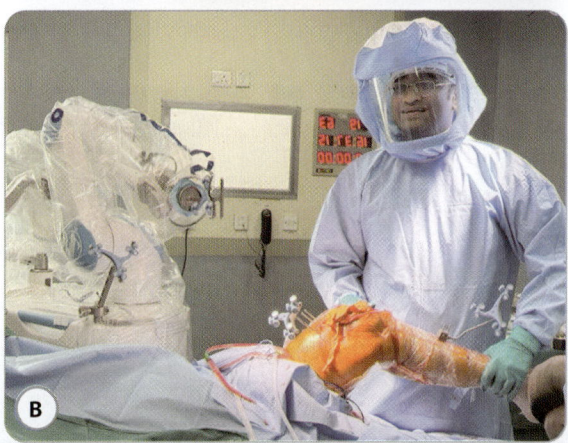

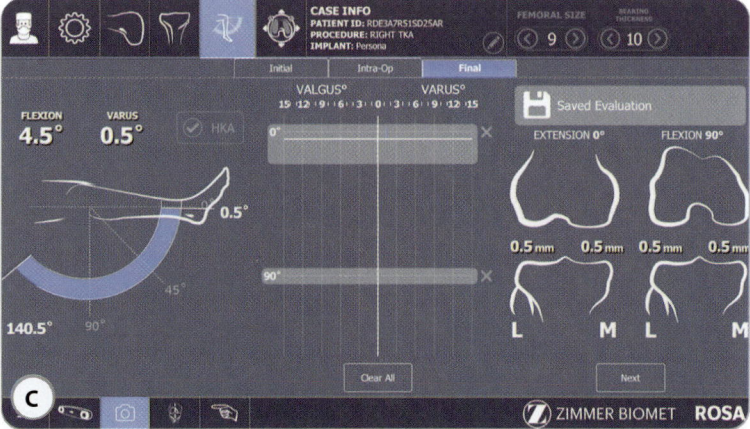

FIGS. 11.33A TO C: (A) Trial implantation done; (B) Clinical picture of checking soft tissue balancing; (C) Trialing and soft tissue balancing confirmation on ROSA system.

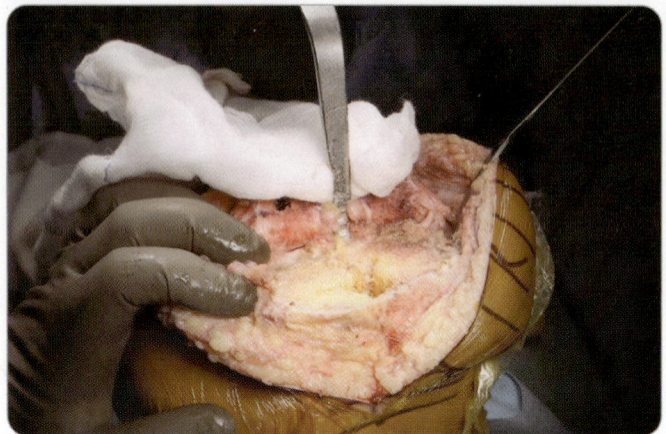

FIG. 11.34A: Proximal tibia prepared with keel slot—ready for tibial component placement.

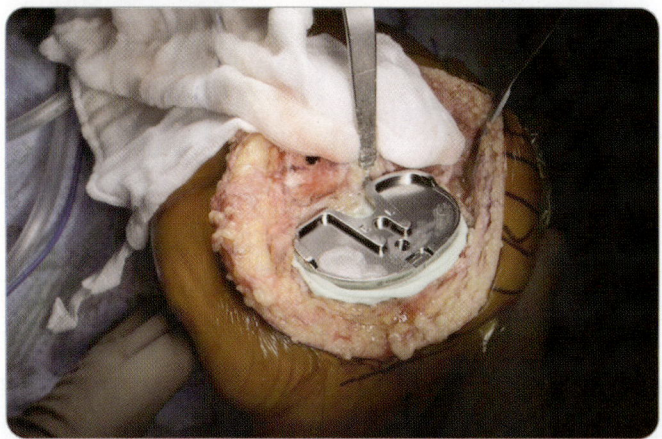

FIG. 11.34B: Final tibial component cemented in position.

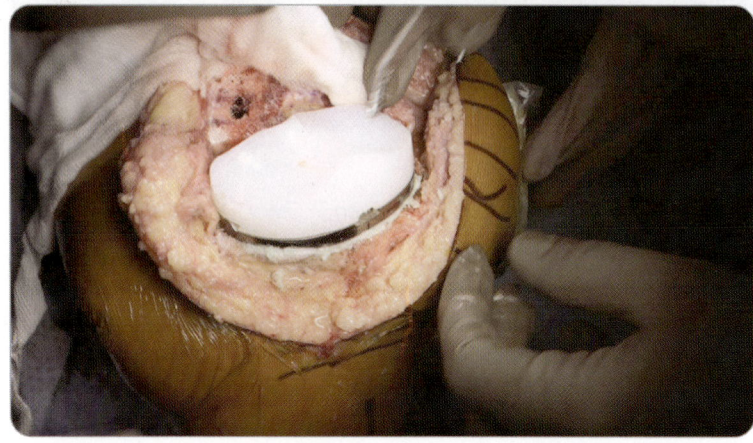

FIG. 11.34C: Final polyethylene insert placed.

CHAPTER 11: ROSA Robotic System

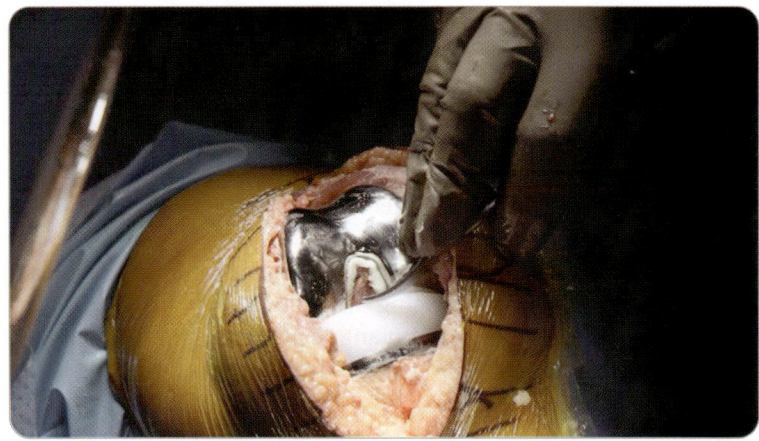

FIG. 11.34D: Final femoral component cemented in position.

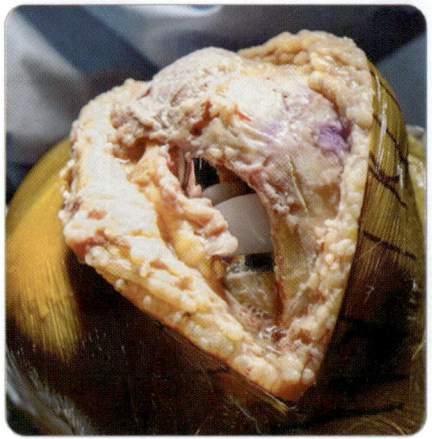

FIG. 11.34E: Patella relocated—final assessment done, knee ready for closure.

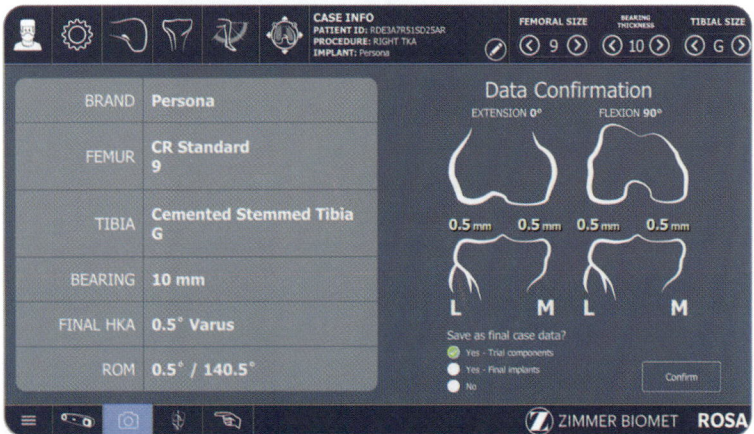

FIG. 11.35: Final kinematic assessment on rosa system.

Radiographic Case Images (Figs. 11.36A to C)

- A 65-year-old female
- C/O: Bilateral knee pain (left > right)

Advantages of ROSA Workflow

- *Surgeon control*: Unlike autonomous robotic systems, ROSA functions as a surgeon-guided tool
- *Real-time adjustments*: Continuous intraoperative feedback enables modifications without preoperative imaging constraints.
- *Improved accuracy*: It enhances implant positioning, gap balancing, and soft tissue preservation, leading to better functional outcomes.

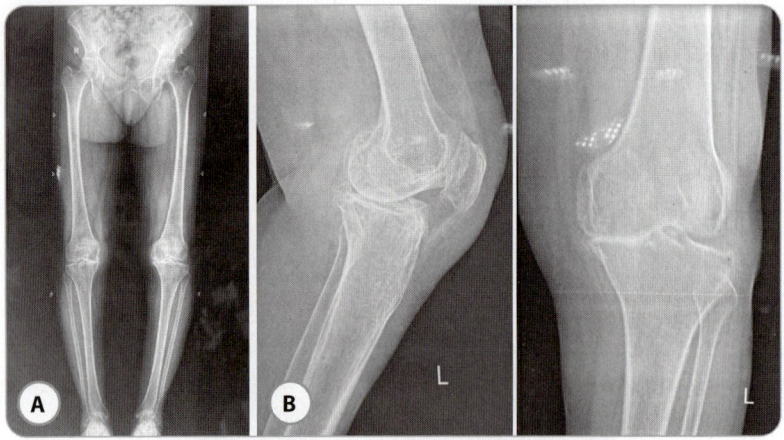

FIGS. 11.36A AND B: (A) Bilateral lower limb scanogram preoperative; (B) Preoperative X-ray left knee anteroposterior/lateral.

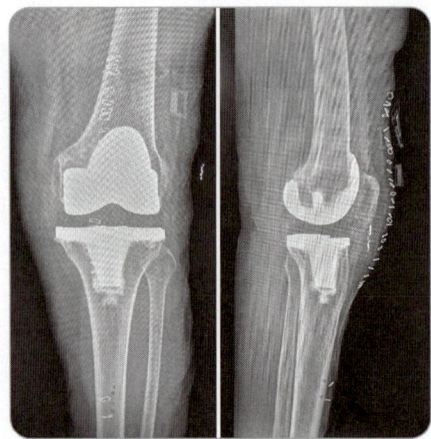

FIG. 11.36C: Postoperative X-ray left knee anteroposterior/lateral.

ACCURACY AND PRECISION IN ROSA NONIMAGE-BASED ROBOTIC TOTAL KNEE REPLACEMENT

Achieving optimal implant alignment and soft tissue balance is critical for long-term success in TKR. The ROSA® Knee System enhances accuracy and precision by utilizing real-time intraoperative data rather than relying on preoperative imaging.

Enhanced Alignment and Implant Positioning

- *Real-time feedback*: ROSA provides real-time feedback on bone cuts, implant positioning, and MA, minimizing human error.
- *Reduced outliers*: Studies have shown reduced outliers in achieving a neutral mechanical axis (≤3° deviation from the ideal 180° alignment).
- *Consistent component positioning*: The system enables consistent femoral and tibial component positioning, reducing complications such as malalignment-related instability or polyethylene wear.

Improved Soft Tissue Balancing

- *Dynamic ligament tension analysis*: Unlike conventional techniques, which rely on manual gap balancing, ROSA analyzes ligament tension dynamically throughout the full range of motion.
- *Real-time gap assessment*: It allows surgeons to optimize soft tissue balance before making final bone cuts.
- *Equal flexion-extension gaps*: Ensures equal flexion-extension gaps, reducing the risk of postoperative stiffness or instability.

Reduced Variability in Surgical Execution

- *Robotic guidance*: It ensures that each step is executed with high precision, reducing intraoperative variability between different surgeons.
- *Customized implant positioning*: Even in cases of severe deformity or bone loss, ROSA adapts intraoperatively, allowing for customized implant positioning.
- *Minimized bone removal*: The use of robotic-assisted bone resection minimizes excessive bone removal, preserving native joint structures.

Clinical Evidence Supporting Accuracy

- *Reduced alignment errors*: Several studies have reported that ROSA achieves more accurate component placement compared to conventional jig-based TKR.
- *Improved functional outcomes*: A 2022 study found that ROSA-assisted TKR reduced alignment errors by up to 50% compared to traditional techniques.
- *Enhanced tibial slope and rotational alignment*: Precision in tibial slope and rotational alignment contributes to improved functional outcomes and patient satisfaction.

Key Benefits of ROSA's Accuracy

- *More precise implant placement*: It reduces risk of early loosening and wear.
- *Better joint kinematics*: It leads to improved range of motion and function.
- *Enhanced soft tissue balance*: It lowers postoperative pain and instability.

BENEFITS OVER TRADITIONAL TECHNIQUES IN ROSA NONIMAGE-BASED ROBOTIC TOTAL KNEE REPLACEMENT

The ROSA® Knee System offers multiple advantages over conventional jig-based and early robotic-assisted TKR techniques. By utilizing real-time intraoperative data and robotic precision without preoperative imaging, ROSA provides benefits in accuracy, efficiency, and patient outcomes.

No Need for Preoperative CT/MRI

- *Cost-effective*: Traditional robotic-assisted TKR often requires CT or MRI scans for preoperative planning, adding extracost and radiation exposure.
- *Radiation-free*: ROSA eliminates this requirement by relying on intraoperative landmark registration and kinematic data, making it more cost-effective and radiation-free.
- *Beneficial for specific patients*: Particularly beneficial for patients with renal impairment or metal implants where CT/MRI may be contraindicated.

Improved Precision with Surgeon Control

- *Reduced variability*: Unlike conventional jigs, which have inherent variability, ROSA provides real-time guidance to ensure accurate bone cuts and implant placement.
- *Surgeon-guided execution*: It maintains full control while utilizing robotic precision for bone resections.

Enhanced Soft Tissue Balancing

- *Optimized ligament tension*: Manual TKR techniques rely on subjective gap balancing, which can lead to asymmetric flexion-extension gaps.
- *Real-time kinematic analysis*: ROSA enables real-time kinematic analysis, optimizing ligament tension, and ensuring proper gap symmetry.
- *Reduced postoperative stiffness*: It results in reduced postoperative stiffness, better knee stability, and improved range of motion.

Reduced Surgical Variability and Learning Curve

- *Standardized workflow*: Traditional TKR outcomes depend heavily on surgeon experience and intraoperative judgment.
- *Reproducible results*: ROSA standardizes the workflow, reducing variability between surgeons, and ensuring reproducible results across different skill levels.

- *Shorter learning curve*: Surgeons experience a shorter learning curve compared to early-generation robotic platforms that require preoperative imaging.

Faster Recovery and Improved Patient Satisfaction
- *Minimized postoperative pain*: More precise bone cuts and soft tissue balance lead to less postoperative pain and swelling.
- *Quicker rehabilitation*: Studies show that patients who undergo ROSA-assisted TKR achieve faster rehabilitation milestones compared to conventional TKR.
- *Higher satisfaction scores*: Improved alignment and kinematics contribute to higher patient-reported satisfaction scores.

Efficiency and Operating Room Workflow Optimization
- *Reduced case time*: By eliminating the preoperative imaging step, ROSA reduces overall case time and logistical complexity.
- *Streamlined process*: Integration of robotic guidance into standard TKR workflows allows for a more streamlined intraoperative process.
- *Shorter surgical times*: Reduced intraoperative adjustments lead to shorter surgical times without compromising accuracy.

Summary of Key Advantages
- *No preoperative imaging required*: Lowers cost and avoids radiation exposure.
- *More precise alignment and bone cuts*: Improves implant longevity.
- *Better soft tissue balance*: Reduces instability and revision rates.
- *Faster recovery and higher patient satisfaction*: Enhanced postoperative outcomes.

CLINICAL OUTCOMES OF ROSA NONIMAGE-BASED ROBOTIC TOTAL KNEE REPLACEMENT

The effectiveness of any surgical innovation is ultimately measured by patient outcomes, complication rates, and implant longevity. ROSA nonimage-based robotic TKR has demonstrated promising results in these areas, offering improved alignment, better functional recovery, and reduced revision rates compared to conventional techniques.

Improved Postoperative Alignment and Implant Longevity
- *Accurate component alignment*: Accurate alignment of components is crucial for reducing wear and preventing early loosening.
- *Reduced deviations*: Studies comparing ROSA-assisted TKR with conventional techniques report lower rates of outliers (>3° deviation) in coronal alignment.
- *Enhanced tibial slope accuracy*: Improved tibial slope accuracy reduces the risk of excessive polyethylene wear.
- *Long-term implant survival*: A 2023 study found that ROSA significantly reduced MA errors, leading to better long-term implant survival.

Faster Functional Recovery

- *Precise bone cuts and soft tissue balance*: Result in early return of mobility and stability.
- *Reduced postoperative pain*: Compared to conventional TKR, ROSA-assisted patients experience less postoperative pain due to minimal soft tissue trauma.
- *Improved functional scores*: Higher Knee Society Scores (KSS) and WOMAC scores at 3 and 6 months postoperatively.

Reduced Complication and Revision Rates

- *Malalignment-related revision rates*: Conventional TKR has a malalignment-related revision rate of 5–10% within the first 10 years.
- *Fewer early complications*: ROSA reduces errors in varus/valgus alignment, rotational mismatch, and tibial slope, all key factors in TKR failure.
- *Multicenter analysis*: Showed that ROSA-assisted TKR had fewer early complications, such as instability and stiffness, compared to traditional methods.

Higher Patient Satisfaction

- *Natural knee kinematics*: Patient-reported outcomes indicate better functional stability and confidence in movement after ROSA-assisted TKR.
- *One-year follow-up*: Higher satisfaction rates (85–90%) due to natural knee kinematics.
- *Reduced dependence on walking aids*: Patients report greater confidence in performing daily activities, leading to improved quality of life.

Long-term Outcomes and Future Prospects

- *Ongoing long-term studies*: While short-term results are promising, long-term studies are ongoing to evaluate implant survival beyond 10–15 years.
- *Future advancements*: Future innovations may further refine ligament balancing algorithms and real-time AI-driven adjustments for even better outcomes.

Summary of Clinical Benefits

- *More precise alignment*: Fewer implant-related complications
- *Better soft tissue balance*: Reduced stiffness and instability
- *Faster rehabilitation*: Shorter hospital stays and improved mobility
- *Higher patient satisfaction*: Improved knee function and quality of life

CHALLENGES AND FUTURE PERSPECTIVES OF ROSA NONIMAGE-BASED ROBOTIC TOTAL KNEE REPLACEMENT

While the ROSA nonimage-based robotic system has significantly improved accuracy, efficiency, and patient outcomes, it still faces certain challenges and limitations. However, ongoing advancements in robotics, artificial intelligence, and surgical techniques are expected to further refine its capabilities.

Challenges in Implementation

- *Learning curve and surgeon adaptation*: Despite its intuitive interface, ROSA still requires surgeon training and adaptation.
    - Familiarization: The shift from conventional to robotic-assisted TKR involves familiarization with robotic workflow and software interface.
    - Real-time adjustments: Adapting to real-time intraoperative adjustments guided by the system.
    - Bone resection techniques: Developing confidence in robotic-assisted bone resection techniques.
    - Proficiency: Studies suggest that after 15–20 cases, surgeons demonstrate proficiency in ROSA-assisted workflows.
- *Cost and resource allocation*: High initial investment in robotic technology may limit accessibility, especially in smaller hospitals.
    - Operational expenses: While ROSA eliminates preoperative imaging costs, operational expenses related to robot maintenance, disposables, and training remain.
    - Cost reduction: Future cost reductions may depend on wider adoption, improved efficiency, and reduced per case costs.
- *Intraoperative technical challenges*: The system relies on accurate anatomical landmark registration.
    - Accurate tracker placement: Inaccurate tracker placement or excessive soft tissue movement may lead to errors in alignment and soft tissue balancing.
    - AI-driven calibration: Advancements in AI-driven intraoperative calibration may improve precision in such cases.

Future Perspectives and Innovations

- *Enhanced AI and machine learning integration*: Future iterations of ROSA could incorporate AI-driven predictive modeling, allowing:
    - Automated soft tissue balance recommendations: Based on real-time intraoperative kinematics
    - Patient-specific gap balancing algorithms: For enhanced ligament tensioning
    - Predictive analytics: For implant longevity and wear patterns
- *Improved haptic feedback and augmented reality (AR) integration*: Future developments may include haptic feedback systems, allowing:
    - Real-time force sensing: During bone resection to prevent overcutting
    - Enhanced visualization: OF ligament tension before final implantation
    - AR overlays: Assisting surgeons by providing 3D real-time alignment data superimposed onto the surgical field
- *Expanding robotic assistance beyond TKR*: The success of ROSA in nonimage-based TKR may pave the way for:
    - Robotic-assisted revision TKR: To manage complex deformities
    - Unicompartmental knee replacement (UKR): Adaptation for hip and shoulder arthroplasty applications

- *Cost reduction and wider accessibility*: Refinement of robotic hardware and disposable components could lead to:
  - Lower per case costs: Making the technology more cost-effective for routine use
  - Compact, mobile systems: Suitable for smaller surgical centers
  - Broader training programs: Reducing the learning curve and increasing adoption across different healthcare settings.

■ CONTRAINDICATIONS

The ROSA Knee System may not be suitable for use in case of:
- Hip pathology with significant bone loss (e.g., avascular necrosis of the femoral head with collapse, severe dysplasia of the femoral head or the acetabulum)
- Hip pathology severely limiting range of motion (e.g., arthrodesis, severe contractures, and chronic severe dislocation)
- Active infections of the knee joint area
- Knee replacement revision surgery
- Presence of strong infrared sources or infrared reflectors in the vicinity of the NavitrackER devices
- Implants that are not compatible with the system
- Contraindications for the implant as given by the implant manufacturer

■ COMPLICATIONS

Possible complications associated with the use of the ROSA Knee System may include but are not limited to the following:
- Infection
- Implant misalignment
- Unstable joint due to erroneous soft tissue balancing

■ CONCLUSION

ROSA nonimage-based robotic TKR represents a significant advancement in precision, alignment, and patient outcomes while eliminating the need for preoperative imaging. However, cost, training requirements, and technical refinements remain challenges. Future innovations, particularly AI-driven planning, enhanced haptic feedback, and AR integration, are expected to further improve its capabilities. As robotic-assisted surgery continues to evolve, ROSA is poised to become a standard tool in personalized knee arthroplasty, ensuring better long-term success and patient satisfaction.

CHAPTER 12

Complication in Robotic Assisted TKA

*Pramod Bhor, Sawankumar Pawar,
Sachin Yashwant Kale, Sourabh Kulkarni*

INTRODUCTION

Total knee arthroplasty has proven to be a reliable treatment option for end-stage degenerative disease. Long-term survivorship rates for total joint arthroplasty are over 95%, according to systematic evaluations. However, national registries show lower survivability rates. Over the past two decades, surgeons have focused on controlling intraoperative variables to improve survival rates. Robotic systems are being used in orthopedic surgery to increase accuracy, reduce outliers, and improve component positioning. Robot-assisted surgery offers numerous benefits, including increased surgical precision and control for surgeons. However, using robotic devices for joint arthroplasty has been linked to risks and complications.

Every orthopedic surgical technique has some level of risk of complications. As a result, it is critical to conduct a comprehensive examination of the issues in order to better comprehend and reduce them. Before this new technology can be extensively employed, it must first be thoroughly evaluated for its complications.

This chapter focuses on the risks and complications associated with robot-assisted surgery, including radiation exposure and pin-related issues, difficulties including registration issues, soft tissue damage, and extended operation hours.

COMMON COMPLICATIONS

Radiation Exposure

Preoperative planning for autonomous and semiautonomous devices is often based on imaging. The CUREXO (autonomous) and MAKO (semiautonomous) systems use preoperative CT scans to produce a 3D map and determine the amount and orientation of bone to be removed.

Radiation dose and biological sensitivity are also important factors to consider. The effective dose (ED) refers to the differential in biological sensitivity and is measured in millisieverts (1 mSv = 1 mGy). According to current literature, single pelvic CT scan typically results in a radiation dosage of roughly 6 mSv and a knee CT results in 1 mSv for adults.

The average radiation exposure for patients in the CT (CUREXO/MAKO protocol) image-based group was 1,135 mGy/cm^2. The average radiation exposure for patients in the [anteroposterior (AP) long leg alignment films (LLAF)] LLAF group was 3,081 Gycm^2. The average radiation exposure for patients undergoing knee AP/lateral and skyline radiographs was the lowest of the categories, at 4.43 Gycm^2. The results between groups were statistically significant when using an ANOVA and posthoc analyses. In this investigation, we discovered a substantial difference in radiation exposure across routine knee radiographs, LLAF, and CT imaging. Nonetheless, the radiation doses for all categories remain within acceptable safety levels.

It is crucial to remember that not all robotic systems carry the same radiation hazards because image-free systems are exempt from this possible disadvantage because they do not need CT scans. It is also critical to remember that CT protocols and technology are always evolving, and that lower dose procedures may be developed in the future to reduce patient risk.

Complications Associated with Pins

Optical arrays, which are fastened to the bone with pins, are used to record the anatomical surface landmarks. A disastrous consequence, however, is a fracture of the femoral or tibial shaft brought on by the pinholes' mechanical weakness. It might be reasonable to take the chance of the stress risers and the resulting mechanical weakness caused by two bicortical pin holes.

Beldame et al. found that the rate of fractures in 385 knees might reach 1.3%. Brown et al. discovered in a more comprehensive meta-analysis that the frequency of fractures through the pin location in the tibia or femur was 0.16%. Obesity and osteoporosis are known patient risk factors for fractures, while the number of drill holes, bigger diameter pins, and bicortical pin insertion were found to be surgical variables.

The diaphysis's bicortical pins provide three primary technical issues. First, the diaphysis may be more vulnerable to fracture than the periarticular bone depends on where the pin holes are located.

Second, it can be challenging to position percutaneous pins precisely in the middle of bone in thighs that are muscular or fat.

Thirdly, the diaphysis becomes weaker when a pin is inserted through both cortices.

The risk of fracture increases more in the bones with the bow, especially femur. Unfortunately percutaneous femoral pin holes are to be made in diaphysis which is at the convexity of the zenith of bow where biomechanical bending forces are maximum.

Precautions

- It might be much better to use a different optical array installation technique that makes the process easier without causing as much bone deterioration. Even strategically positioned pin holes in the diaphysis seem to inherently

reduce the bone's mechanical strength. Whenever possible it is preferable to place array pins within the metaphyseal bone where bending and torsional forces are minimal. Consequently, the placement of optical array pins within the metaphyseal bone is crucial **(Figs. 12.1A and B)**.
- Try to avoid putting bicortical pins. Instead use near bicortical or one and half cortical technique. In this technique, the surgeon has to take purchase of the first cortex then reach the opposite cortex and abutt tip on the inner cortex.

Management

A distinct pattern of pin-site fractures in which fractures happen on average 12.6 weeks following arthroplasty. Prior to fracture events, patients reported experiencing peculiar thigh pain for a few days. These fractures were treated with intramedullary treatment or periprosthetic plates and were linked to mild or indirect trauma **(Figs. 12.2A to C)**.

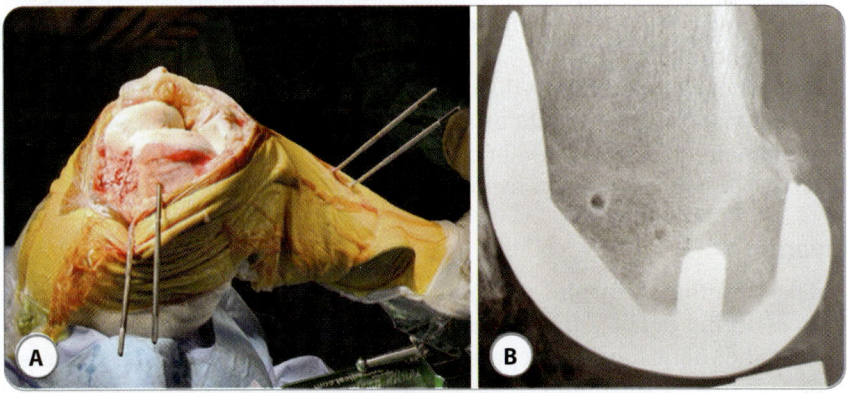

FIGS. 12.1A AND B: A lateral X-ray of total knee arthroplasty (TKA) shows the position of the pin hole after periarticular femoral pin placement.

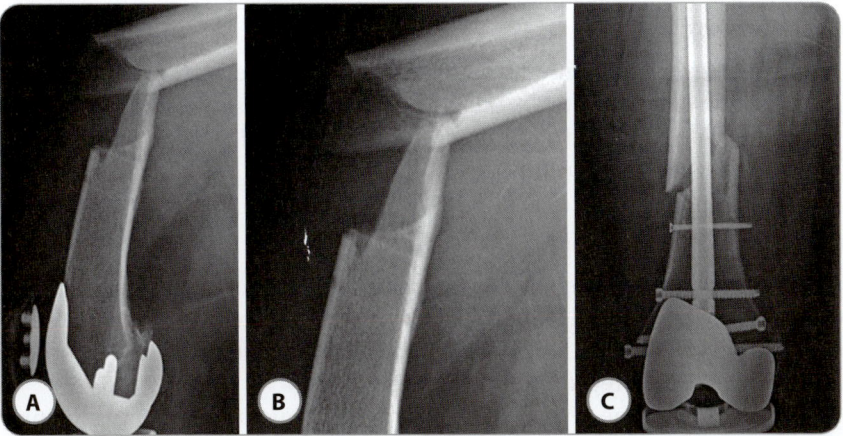

FIGS. 12.2A TO C: (A) A lateral X-ray shows a short oblique periprosthetic femoral fracture. (B) A close-up view shows the fracture originated from the stress riser left by the diaphyseal pin hole. (C) An anteroposterior X-ray shows the fracture is fixed with intramedullary femoral rodding.

The minor pin-site complications such as bleeding, suture abscess, and neuropraxia can be managed conservatively.
- Immediate identification of fracture using intraoperative imaging
- Stabilization with nail, screws, plates, or cerclage wires
- Adjust the surgical approach to ensure proper fixation and prevent further damage
- Postoperative care includes restricted weight-bearing and regular imaging to monitor healing.

Soft Tissue Injuries

One of the most feared complications in arthroplasty is iatrogenic soft tissue injuries including patellar tendon rupture, popliteus muscle injury, medial collateral ligament (MCL) injury, and injury to popliteal neurovascular bundle. Majorly these injuries happen when:
- Error in preoperative or precut planning
- Intraoperatively array pins have moved, displacing bone markers after bone registration. Hence, the spatial orientation of bone changes with respect to the robotic arm.
- If the robot cart marker gets displaced while fixing the robot for bone cutting.

It is still not possible for robotic systems to make original choices or alter the preprogrammed path in the event of an unforeseen circumstance. The surgeon might have to switch back to conventional methods in certain situations.

Prevention

- Make sure that array pins will not get displaced by either direct or indirect forces during gap balancing or during positioning of limb for cutting.
- While the robotic tool is preparing the bone surface, it is crucial to preserve the soft tissues surrounding the milling or cutting area. Always be vigilant when cutting is going on.
- While doing preplanning, always consider looking at the cutting path.

Management

- Immediate repair of injured structures using sutures or grafts.
- Application of intraoperative imaging to ensure no residual damage.
- Postoperative immobilization followed by a tailored rehabilitation protocol focusing on gradual range-of-motion exercises.

Registration Malfunctions

Robot-assisted surgery depends on accurate registration, which is reliant on the anatomy of the patient as well as the design of markers, arrays, and pins. As demonstrated by Hausmann et al., the landmark pointing approach and soft tissue thickness affect registration accuracy.

Using an image-free system has a risk of inadequate preoperative planning and the inability to use a 3D digital map to confirm the anatomic registration landmarks during operation. Thus, in patients with aberrant anatomy, CT-based systems may still offer certain benefits over imageless systems.

Reregistration is required in the unavoidable event of registration errors in order to complete the process and meet system criteria. This could lengthen the surgical operation and, in the event that the fault cannot be fixed, could even result in a switch to conventional treatments.

Another reason for registration error is due to remaining cartilage thickness on the less affected side. In image-based systems, complete penetration of cartilage by the pointed tip of the registration probe is compulsory. Tip of the probe must rest against the cortical bone while registration.

Calibration Errors or Software Glitches

In such case following measures can be taken:
- Pause the procedure to recalibrate the robotic system.
- If unresolved, switch to conventional manual techniques.
- Notify the manufacturer to investigate and prevent recurrence.

CONCLUSION

While robotic knee arthroplasty offers numerous advantages, complications can occur and require timely, evidence-based management. A proactive approach encompassing prevention, early detection, and tailored interventions is essential to maximize surgical outcomes and improve patient satisfaction. Through ongoing advancements in robotic technology and surgical techniques, the rate of complications continues to decline, paving the way for even better patient care and outcome.

CHAPTER 13

Advantages of Robotic Total Knee Replacement

*Pramod Bhor, Sawankumar Pawar, Sachin Yashwant Kale,
Sourabh Kulkarni, Shivam Mehra*

■ INTRODUCTION

Robotic-assisted surgery is one revolutionary advancement in total knee replacement (TKR) that has been made over the years. Despite major improvements in implant design, materials, and patient-specific rehabilitation protocols, up to 20% of patients report dissatisfaction following total knee arthroplasty (TKA). Limb alignment and precise implant placement are widely regarded as the most important predicting variables for long-term implant longevity, patient fulfilment, and clinical outcomes. Robotic-assisted TKR improves patient outcomes, accuracy, and problem-solving when compared to conventional methods. This chapter discusses in detail the primary advantages of robotic TKR, which include enhanced long-term outcomes, less soft tissue damage, individualized surgical planning, enhanced precision, and faster recovery.

Increased Surgical Accuracy

One of the most important benefits of robotic-assisted TKR is its improved accuracy. Traditional TKR depends majorly on surgeon's expertise and manual alignment methods, which could introduce variation. On the other hand, robotic systems guarantee precise bone cuts and implant placement by means of sophisticated imaging, intraoperative mapping, and real-time feedback. This level of accuracy is vital for best results

Best Alignment

Various alignment strategies differ from each other depending on femoral and tibial varus/valgus in few degrees of angular variation and submillimeter depth of bone cutting. Robotic systems allow measured variations in cutting of bone with submillimeter accuracy. Hence, placement of the femoral and tibial components can have exact measured and reproducible variation in degrees and millimeters. Therefore, robotics can allow surgeons to use different alignment strategies with precision.

Balanced Soft Tissues

As optical tracking systems provide real-time feedback of medial/lateral gap values in millimeters, robotics enables surgeons to get a well-balanced knee, which is crucial for stability and lifespan.

Reproducibility

Due to submillimeter accuracy of cutting and repetition of cut accuracy of >0.5 mm, robotic systems can reproduce the same results among various patients by reducing intersurgeon variance and human error.

CUSTOM PREOPERATIVE PLANNING

Advanced preoperative planning using CT scans, or intraoperative imaging, is included in robotic TKR.

The system customizes the operation depending on the particular anatomy of each patient, therefore, enhancing implant fit and biomechanics. Surgeons may select the most ideal alignment by first modeling several implant positions and then making any bone incisions.

MINIMIZED SOFT TISSUE DAMAGE

The robotic system assists to keep natural soft tissue balance, therefore lessening postoperative stiffness and enhancing early functional results by limiting interference to muscles and tendons.

LESS BLOOD LOSS

Conventional TKR depends on the intramedullary rod, which can cause intramedullary bleeding. As robotic assisted TKR doesn't need intramedullary rod insertion bleeding is minimized. Also minimal soft tissue release due to robotic-assisted gap balancing leads to less bleeding. Studies have indicated that robotic-assisted TKR decreases perioperative bleeding, therefore reducing the need of postoperative complications and blood transfusions.

BONE CONSERVATION

The robotic system removes only the necessary bone, thanks to preemptive gap balancing and precision of cutting with the help of robotic cutting tools.

FASTER REHABILITATION AND RECOVERY

Robotic-assisted TKR accelerates and improves recovery owing to minimal soft tissue release, lesser manipulation of leg while cutting, lesser blood loss, better alignment, conservative bone cuts, and exact implant positioning.

Early mobilization lets patients start physiotherapy sooner since they suffer lower pain and swelling.

Many experiments indicate that patients with robotic TKR spend *less time in hospital* than those undergoing alternative TKR.

Patients recover knee functionality faster, so they can get back to daily work sooner.

LESS RISK OF COMPLICATIONS IN SURGERY[4,10]

Robotic TKR lowers the risk associated with conventional TKR including:
- *Malalignment-related failures*: Accurate implant placement reduces risk of instability, abnormal wear, and implant loosening.
- Blood loss and transfusion related complications
- *Pulmonary embolism* is less expected due to avoidance of intramedullary rod insertion.

BETTER PATIENT SATISFACTION AND LONG-TERM RESULTS

Robotic-assisted TKR leads to better patient satisfaction and long-term results. Majorly due to perfect patient-specific implant placement, minimal soft tissue release, less blood loss, less pain, faster recovery, and increase longevity of TKR.

SURGEON'S BENEFITS

Although robotic TKR necessitates initial training, doctors can benefit from it in the long run:
- *Improved intraoperative feedback*: Surgeons can make better choices during the procedure thanks to real-time data.
- *Fatigue reduction*: By helping the surgeon make accurate bone cuts, the robotic technology lessens the physical strain on the surgeon. In active systems, physical burden is significantly reduced.

CONCLUSION

Robotic-assisted TKR has transformed knee replacement surgery by increasing accuracy, lowering complications, and improving patient outcomes. With advantages such as improved implant placement, less soft tissue damage, faster recovery, and lower revision rates, robotic TKR is the future of knee arthroplasty. As technology advances, robotic devices will improve surgical techniques, providing even more benefits to both patients and surgeons.

CHAPTER 14

Rehabilitation in Robotic-guided Knee Arthroplasty

Sagar Deshpande, Sachin Yashwant Kale, Pramod Bhor, Sushant Srivastava, Sachiti Sachin Kale, Siddhant Pramod Bhor

INTRODUCTION

Knee osteoarthritis (KOA) is a chronic degenerative condition that primarily affects the articular cartilage in the knee joint. Although KOA is most common in older adults, it can also affect younger individuals, particularly those who have experienced trauma or undergone surgery. The classic symptoms of KOA include pain and functional limitations, which, in severe cases, can lead to joint deformity and significantly impair mobility. Decision-making for knee arthroplasty is guided by radiographic severity and the degree of functional impairment caused by persistent pain, swelling, irreversible stiffness, and structural deformities, all of which can drastically reduce quality of life. Although traditional knee arthroplasty methods have shown great long-term results, issues such as implant malalignment, soft tissue imbalance, and patient dissatisfaction remain. Recently, robotics-assisted knee arthroplasty (RAKA) has emerged as a promising development designed to improve surgical precision, optimize implant placement, and enhance functional outcomes. Common robotic platforms used in knee arthroplasty include the MAKO robotic-arm system, ROSA knee system, NAVIO surgical system, and OMNI Botics. While each system offers distinct features, they all share the same objective of improving surgical precision and patient outcomes. Robotic-guided knee arthroplasty has gained widespread popularity in recent years due to its superior outcomes and quicker recovery times. Robotic systems in knee arthroplasty use preoperative imaging (such as CT scans or image-free intraoperative mapping) to generate a personalized 3D model of the knee. This model facilitates precise planning for implant placement and ligament balancing before any bone is altered. During the procedure, robotic technology aids the surgeon by regulating the depth, angle, and position of bone cuts, ensuring higher accuracy and minimizing errors that can occur with manual methods. This advanced surgical approach offers increased precision, personalized implant placement, and improved tissue balance, potentially leading to faster healing and a reduced risk of complications. As a result, many patients experience a quicker return to normal activities. Additionally, robotic knee surgeries often incorporate enhanced recovery after surgery (ERAS) protocols, which prioritize patient health by ensuring adequate nutritional support, effective pain management, proper fluid and hydration levels, and promoting early mobilization. Tailored preoperative and postoperative rehabilitation protocols are essential in maximizing the benefits of robotic knee arthroplasty, leading to improved surgical outcomes, faster recovery, and long-term joint functions as they significantly impact the overall success and recovery of the patient. Programs are implemented following surgery to optimize recovery and minimize hospital stays. Preoperative rehabilitation for total knee arthroplasty (TKA), particularly with robotic-assisted surgery, is designed to optimize the patient's condition before surgery to ensure better outcomes, faster recovery, and more efficient rehabilitation postsurgery. Robotics in TKA allows for greater precision during the surgical procedure, but preoperative rehabilitation remains a crucial part of preparing the body and mind for the procedure. The postoperative period is also a critical phase in the recovery process, requiring patience, dedication to rehabilitation, and vigilant monitoring for complications. Most patients experience significant pain relief and increased mobility, with the healing of the knee joint progressing steadily over time. Achieving long-term recovery depends on a personalized physical therapy regimen, lifestyle modifications, and ongoing monitoring. The physical therapy protocol is designed to restore joint mobility, strengthen the surrounding muscles, and optimize functional outcomes. Rehabilitation is typically structured into phases, each with specific objectives and interventions. The precise protocol will vary depending on the surgeon's recommendations and the unique needs of the individual patient. This comprehensive rehabilitative approach integrating cutting-edge surgical techniques, ERAS protocols, and individualized rehabilitation provides patients with the best possible opportunity for a successful and rapid recovery following robotic knee arthroplasty.

The following rehabilitation preoperative protocol can be used in minimally invasive robotic knee arthroplasty **(Table 14.1)**.

TABLE 14.1: Preoperative rehabilitation protocol for minimally invasive robotic knee arthroplasty.

Phases of rehabilitation	Goals of rehabilitation	Rehabilitation minimally invasive robotic knee arthroplasty
Preoperative phase (3–4 weeks)	• Patient education and counseling • Weight management • Diet and nutrition • Pain management • Flexibility and range of motion training • Strengthening exercises for muscle memory	*Patient education and counseling*: • Understanding robotic knee arthroplasty • Indications and benefits • Preoperative preparation • Surgical procedure explanation • Postoperative expectations • Recovery timeline • Potential risks and complication • Long-term outcomes and follow-up • Addressing patient concerns

Continued

Continued

Phases of rehabilitation	Goals of rehabilitation	Rehabilitation minimally invasive robotic knee arthroplasty

	• Low threshold balance and proprioceptive training
	• Exercises and techniques for respiratory and circulatory maintenance
	• Cardiovascular fitness training
	• Re-education of bed transfer and gait training
		Weight management:
		• Balanced diet
		• Regular exercise
		• Monitor portion size
		• Hydration
		• Avoid quick weight loss
		Diet and nutrition:
		• Protein rich food
		• Anti-inflammatory food
		• Calcium and vitamin D
		• Avoid complex carbohydrates
		• Healthy fats
		• Maintain hydration
		• Limit process food and sugar
		Pain management:
		• *Modalities*:
		  ○ Ice pack for 15–20 minutes
		  ○ Shock wave
		  ○ Matrix rhythm therapy for quadriceps **(Fig. 14.1)**, hamstrings **(Fig. 14.2)**, and calf **(Fig. 14.3)**
		  ○ Low intensity class III LASER **(Fig. 14.4)**
		  ○ Neuromuscular electrical stimulation (NMES)
		• *Soft tissue release*:
		  ○ MFR (myofascial release)
		Flexibility and range of motion training:
		• Quadriceps stretch—wall or chair supported standing active stretch, prone knee bending Passive stretch **(Fig. 14.5)**
		• Hamstring stretch—chair or low stool standing toe touch active stretch **(Fig. 14.6)**, long sitting pulls active stretch
		• Calf stretch—heel drop active stretch on stairs or wall
		• Hip flexors stretch—half kneeling hip flexor active stretch
		• IT band stretch—standing cross leg active stretch and with foam roller

Continued

Continued

Phases of rehabilitation	Goals of rehabilitation	Rehabilitation minimally invasive robotic knee arthroplasty
		Low threshold Strengthening exercises for muscle memory: • Isometric exercise for quadriceps (**Fig. 14.7**), hamstring (**Fig. 14.8**), and gluteal in supine • Core strengthening exercises—TA activation • Open chain exercises (OCE) SLR (**Fig. 14.9**), side lying hip abduction (**Fig. 14.10**), and extension • Active heel slides • Active dynamic quadriceps sets • Upper extremity strengthening regimen • Close chain exercises (CCE) wall squats, forwards lunges *Balance and proprioception training*: • Weight shifting • Single-leg stance (**Fig. 14.11**) • Tandem stance—heel-to-toe standing • Heel-to-toe walking—tandem walking • Balance and on proprioception—wobble board or balance board exercise • Bosu ball (**Fig. 14.12**) or foam pad balance training • Functional reach exercise • Single-leg clock taps • Lateral step up-down (**Fig. 14.13**) and forward step up-down (**Fig. 14.14**) • Walking on uneven surfaces • Perturbation training *Gait training*: • Weight shifting exercises • Heel-to-toe walking • Marching on place • Stair climbing practice • Walking on different terrains • Obstacle navigation *Exercises and techniques for respiratory and breathing exercises and chest physiotherapy*: • Diaphragmatic breathing • Thoracic expansion • Pursed lip • Segmental expansion exercise • Huffing-coughing • Incentive spirometry *Exercises and technique for circulatory maintenance*: • Ankle pump • Toe taps foot circle • DVT stocking • Compression bandaging and elevation

Continued

Continued

Phases of rehabilitation	Goals of rehabilitation	Rehabilitation minimally invasive robotic knee arthroplasty
		Cardiovascular fitness training: • Static cycling **(Fig. 14.15)** • Treadmill walking **(Fig. 14.16)** • Elliptical training • Aquatic training • Upper body ergometer *Reeducation of bed transfer*: Supine > bridging > side lying > edge of bed > rocking movement > reach out > standing > chair sitting

(ATM: ankle toe movement; DVT: deep vein thrombosis; CCE: close chain exercises; NMES: neuromuscular electrical stimulation; TA: transversus abdominis; SLR: straight leg raise; OCE: open chain exercises)

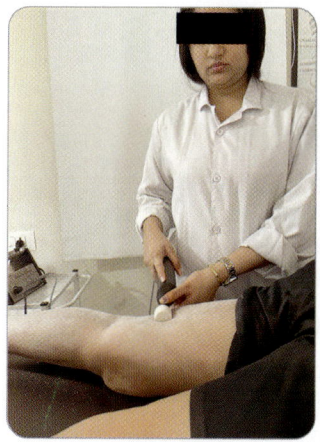

FIG. 14.1: Matrix therapy for hamstrings.

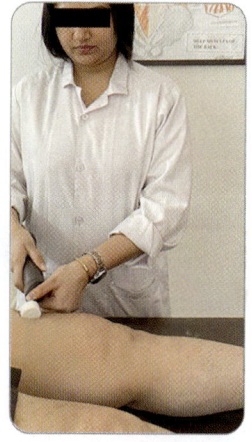

FIG. 14.2: Matrix therapy for quadriceps.

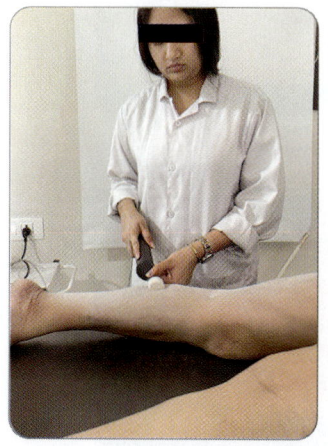

FIG. 14.3: Matrix therapy for calf.

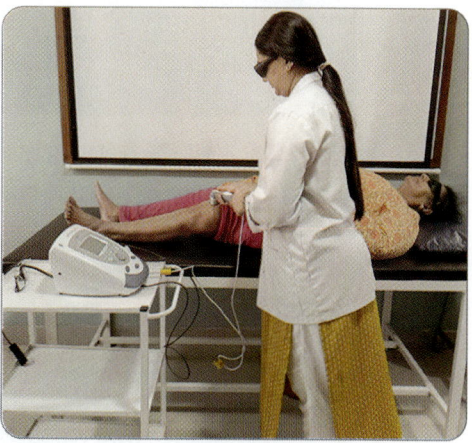

FIG. 14.4: Low-intensity class III LASER.

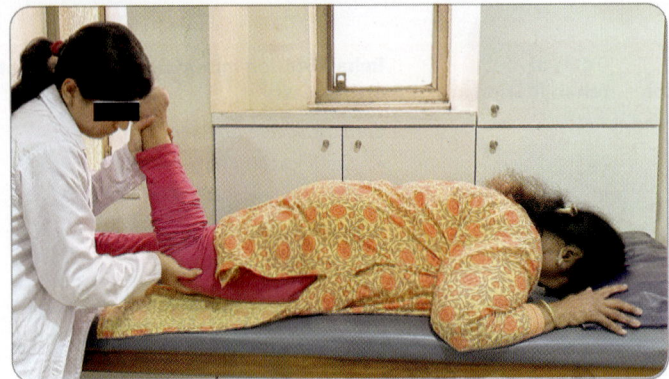

FIG. 14.5: Quadriceps stretch (passive).

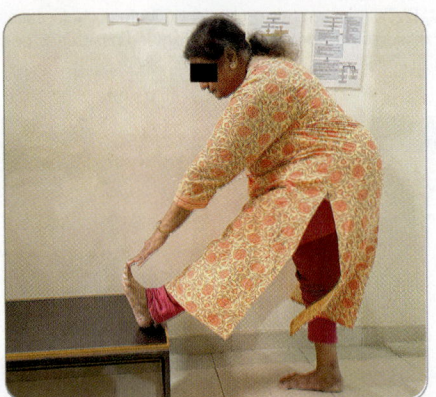

FIG. 14.6: Hamstring stretch (active).

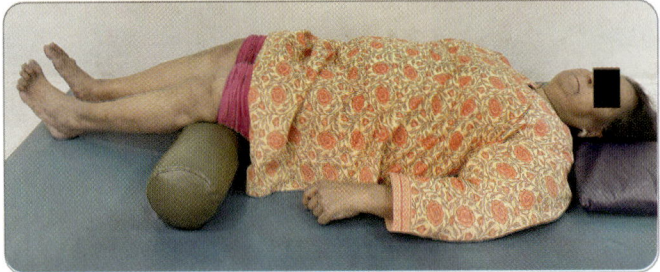

FIG. 14.7: Static quadriceps (isometrics).

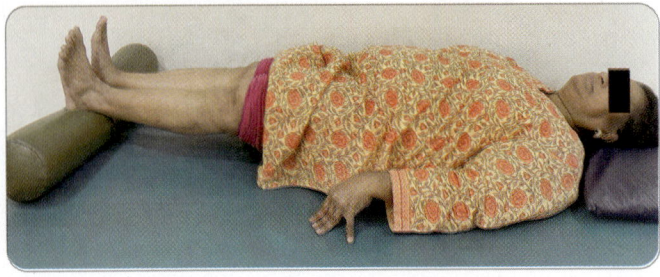

FIG. 14.8: Static hamstring (isometrics).

CHAPTER 14: Rehabilitation in Robotic-guided Knee Arthroplasty

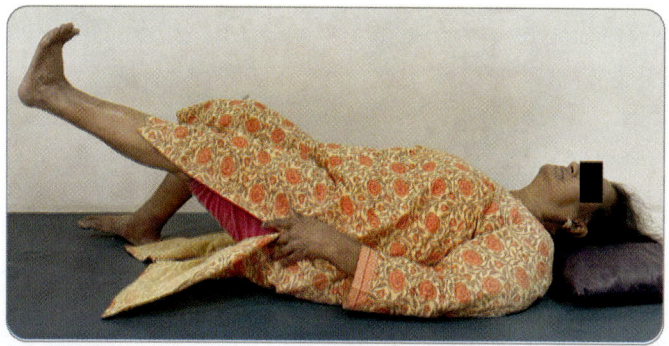

FIG. 14.9: Straight leg raise (SLR) (without weight cuff).

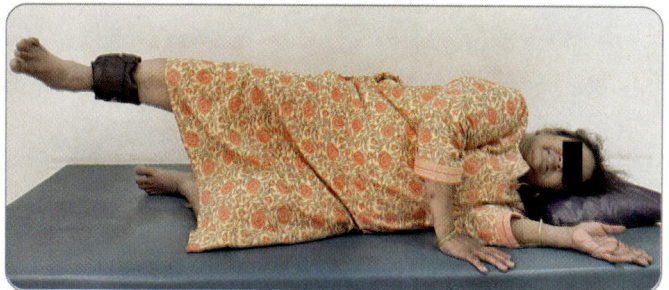

FIG. 14.10: Hip abduction (without weight cuff).

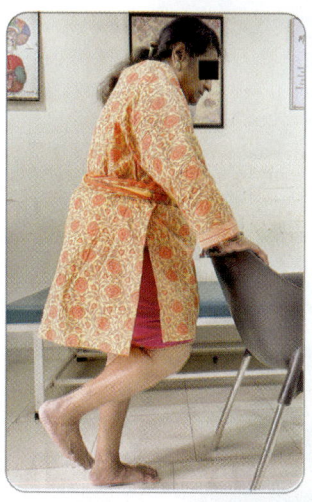

FIG. 14.11: Single leg stance (with support).

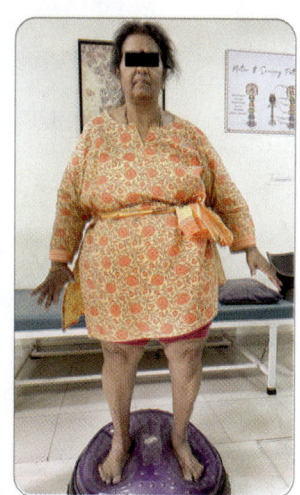

FIG. 14.12: Balancing on Bosu ball.

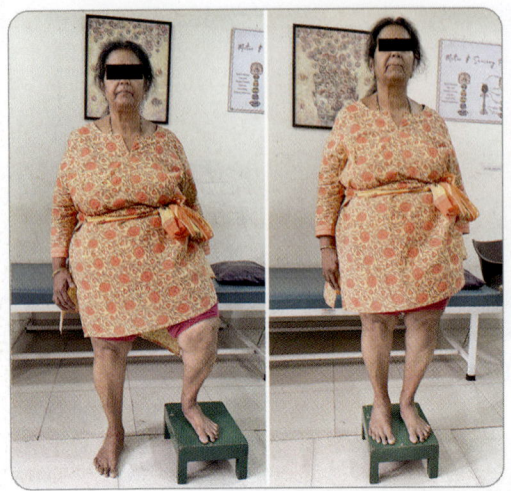

FIG. 14.13: Step up-step down (lateral).

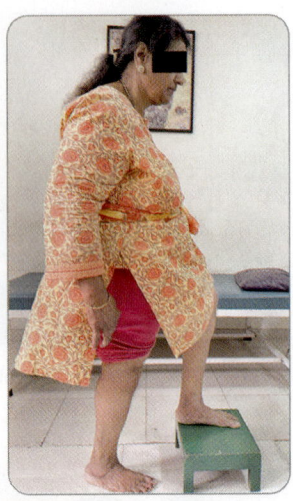

FIG. 14.14: Step up-step down (forward).

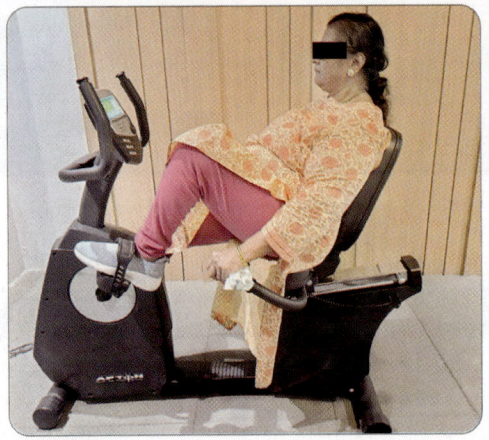

FIG. 14.15: Cycling.

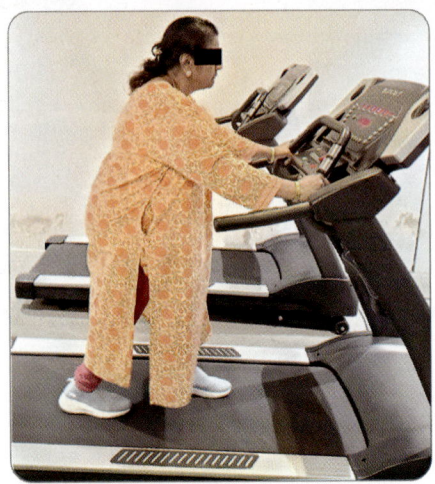

FIG. 14.16: Treadmill walking.

The following rehabilitation postoperative protocol can be used in minimally invasive robotic knee arthroplasty **(Table 14.2)**.

TABLE 14.2: Postoperative rehabilitation protocol for minimally invasive robotic knee arthroplasty.

Phases of rehabilitation	Goals of rehabilitation	Rehabilitation minimally invasive robotic knee arthroplasty
Immediate postoperative phase (0–2 weeks)	• Patient counseling • Protection of the implant and suture site • Minimize pain and swelling • Prevent extension lag at knee • Postoperative wound care • Prevent arthrogenic muscle inhibition • Achieve adequate quadriceps contraction • Prevent muscle shortening and guarding • Bed transfer • Initiate early weight bearing and gait training with a walking aid • Prevent immediate postoperative complications	*Mobility*: • Ankle pumps (ATM) **(Fig. 14.17)** • DVT stocking, elevation of leg with ATM on elevation pillow for swelling reduction • Supine AAROM heel slides • Supine gastrocnemius/soleus mild stretch • Knee PROM to AROM (0–40°) • Passive to active VMO activation • Hip mobility exercises—SLR **(Fig. 14.9)**, hip abduction **(Fig. 14.10)** • Soft tissue manipulation to quadriceps, hamstrings, and calf • Edge of bed sitting • Sit-to-stand transfer training (commode training) • Protective early full weight bearing with walking aid and close supervision **(Fig. 14.18)** *Strengthening*: • Static quadriceps **(Fig. 14.7)**, hamstrings sets **(Fig. 14.8)** • Core strengthening exercises—TA activation • Short angle active dynamic quadriceps sets • Hip strengthening—static gluteal sets, short hip flexor activation sets • Upper extremity strengthening regimen *Modality*: • Cryotherapy for 15–20 minutes around knee joint • Neuromuscular electrical stimulation (NMES) for muscle contraction • Continuous passive movement for knee (0–70° as per tolerance) *Prerequisites for progression*: • Minimal pain and swelling around knee • No extension lag in knee • Knee AROM ≥ 90° • Independent transfers and ambulation at least 100 feet with appropriate assistive device and close supervision • SLR without extension lag in knee

Continued

Continued

Phases of rehabilitation	Goals of rehabilitation	Rehabilitation minimally invasive robotic knee arthroplasty
Intermediate postoperative phase (2–4 weeks)	• Continue implant protection • Minimize pain and swelling • Prevent extension lag at knee • Improve knee range and patella mobility • Improve neuromuscular control • Improve muscle flexibility • Improve quadriceps and hamstring strength • Improve knee proprioception • Improve joint stability • Initiate open-chain exercises (OCE) and progress to close-chain exercises (CCE) • Progress with gait training	*Mobility*: Continue phase 1 exercises: • Soft tissue mobilization around knee joint • Prone hangs to prevent extension lag • Patellar mobilization—medial-lateral glide (**Fig. 14.19**), superior-inferior glide (**Fig. 14.20**) • Knee PROM to AROM 0–90° • Initiate gentle hamstring stretch and posterior capsule stretch in supine, quadriceps stretch in prone • Initiate active VMO activation • Supine active heel slides and seated long angle quadriceps • Initiate OCE in standing-hamstring curls, Forward hip knee flexion, hip abduction with weight (**Fig. 14.21**) • Forward–backward waking, side walking, zig-zag walking • Static cycling without resistance (**Fig. 14.15**) • Initiate step up-down, lateral (**Fig. 14.13**) and forward (**Fig. 14.14**) with support 2–4-inch stepper • Staircase climbing with support • Walking without support but with close supervision *Strengthening*: • Initiate supine double leg bridging • SLR with hold • Hip extensor, abductor, strengthening with hold • Multiangle VMO activation with hold • Progression in TA activation exercises • Multiple angle isometrics to quadriceps in sitting (e.g., 90°, 60°, and 30°) • Initiate mini wall squats with support (0–45°) • Balance training with a bilateral stance • Obstacle walking with close supervision *Modality*: • Cryotherapy for 15–20 minutes • Biofeedback/electrical stimulation • Matrix rhythm therapy for quadriceps (**Fig. 14.2**), hamstrings (**Fig. 14.1**), and calf (**Fig. 14.3**)

Continued

Continued

Phases of rehabilitation	Goals of rehabilitation	Rehabilitation minimally invasive robotic knee arthroplasty
		Prerequisites for progression: • No pain and swelling • Knee AROM ≥ 110° • Improved both quadriceps and hamstring strength • Walking without support • Improved patella mobility • Independent transfers and ambulation at least 100 feet without support close supervision • 1 staircase flight climbing without support
Late postoperative phase (4–6 weeks)	• Maintain muscle flexibility • Improve motor control • Improve proprioception and balance • Maintain joint stability • Improve quadriceps and hamstring strength • Progression of closed-chain exercises • Progress with gait training • Improve cardiovascular strength	*Mobility*: • Continue phase 1 and phase 2 exercises: • Knee PROM to AROM (0–125°) • Patellar mobilization with quadriceps activation (medial-lateral glide—**Fig. 14.19**), (superior-inferior glide—**Fig. 14.20**) • Soft tissue mobilization around knee joint • Initiate CCE forward and lateral lunges • IT band stretch/ foam roller, standing hamstring stretch **(Fig. 14.8)** • Supine CCE bilateral bridging with hold, initiate unilateral bridging • step-up, step-down, and lateral step-up exercises with ankle weight and support (up to 8 inch) • Forward and backward, side, and zigzag walking with ankle weights • Supervised obstacle walking with ankle weights • Walking without support and close supervision • Staircase climbing with support *Strengthening*: • Multiple angle quadriceps strengthening in sitting with progressive weights, e.g., 90° **(Fig. 14.22)**, 60° **(Fig. 14.23)**, 30°, and TheraBand (e.g., 90°, 60°, and 30°) • Prone and standing multi angle hamstrings curls with progressive weights **(Fig. 14.24)** and TheraBand. e.g., 90°, 60°, and 30° • Multi angle VMO activation with weights **(Fig. 14.25)** • SLR with weight **(Fig. 14.26)** • Hip extensor strengthening with weights **(Fig. 14.27)**

Continued

Continued

Phases of rehabilitation	Goals of rehabilitation	Rehabilitation minimally invasive robotic knee arthroplasty
		• Initiate mini squats with support (0–90) • Static cycling with progressive resistance **(Fig. 14.15)** • Core strengthening • Balance training on an unstable surface—foam mat, stability board, and Bosu ball **(Fig. 14.12)** • Balance with perturbation • Initiate treadmill walking with supervision **(Fig. 14.16)** *Modality:* • Cryotherapy for 15–20 minutes • Aquatic therapy • Matrix rhythm therapy for quadriceps muscle **(Fig. 14.2)**, hamstrings muscle **(Fig. 14.1)**, and calf muscle **(Fig. 14.3)** *Prerequisites for progression:* • No pain or signs of active swelling with inflammation • Knee AROM up to 130° • Improved quadriceps and hamstring strength • No compensation in squat • Unilateral stance for 20–30 seconds • Independent transfers and ambulation at least 200 feet without support and close supervision • One staircase flight climbing without support and supervision
Return to activity/function phase (≥12 weeks)	• Maintain knee proprioception • Improve muscle strength and endurance • Improve balance and coordination • Improve aerobic ability fitness • Improve neuromuscular control • Improve maximum muscle torque strength and endurance • Load absorption training	Continue phase three exercises *Mobility:* • Knee PROM-AROM (0–135°) • Recumbent bicycling with resistance **(Fig. 14.15)** • Balance and proprioception training on an unstable surface—foam mats, Bosu ball, and wobble board **(Fig. 14.12)** • Balance and proprioception training unpredictable surfaces (community dwelling, e.g., garden and parks) • Mild-to-moderate forward, backward, and side hopping • Walking on a treadmill with progressive speed **(Fig. 14.16)** • Retrograde walking on a treadmill *Strengthening:* • Body weight squats • Single leg squat • Closed chain core strengthening exercises

(AROM: active range of motion; AAROM: active-assisted range of motion; ATM: ankle-toe movement; CCE: close chain exercises; IT: iliotibial; MFR: myofascial release; NMES: neuromuscular electrical stimulation; PROM: passive range of motion; SLR: straight leg raise; TA: transversus abdominis; OCE: open chain exercises; VMO: vastus medialis obliquus)

CHAPTER 14: Rehabilitation in Robotic-guided Knee Arthroplasty | 197

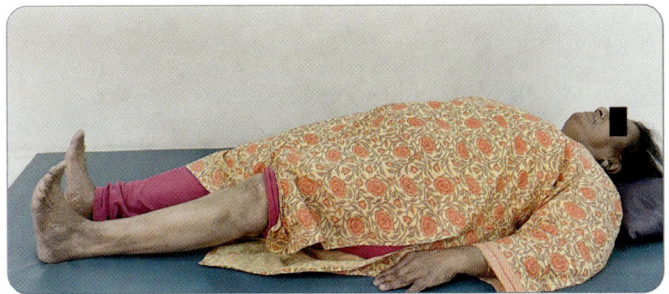

FIG. 14.17: Ankle–toe pumps (ATMs).

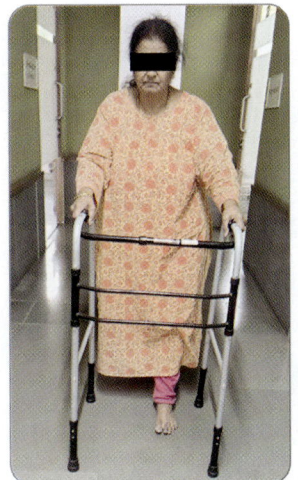

FIG. 14.18: Full weight bearing with walker.

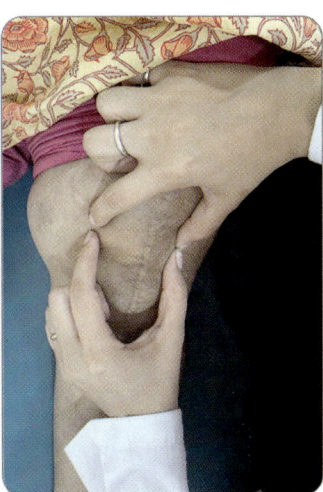

FIG. 14.19: Patellar Mobilization (medial-lateral).

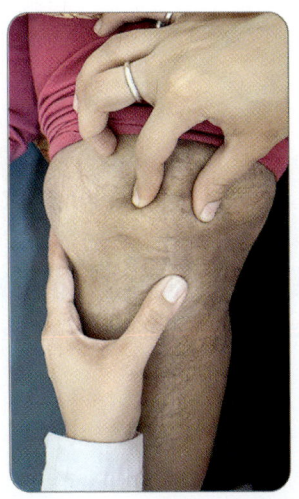

FIG. 14.20: Patellar mobilization (superior-inferior).

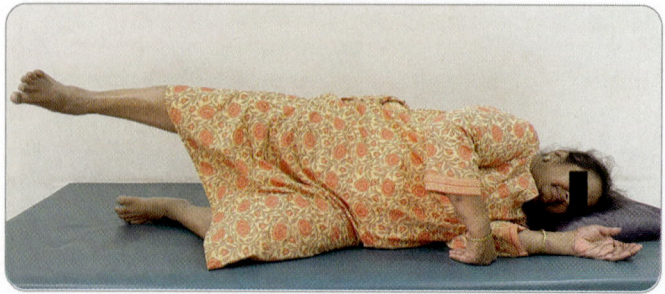

FIG. 14.21: Hip abduction (without weight).

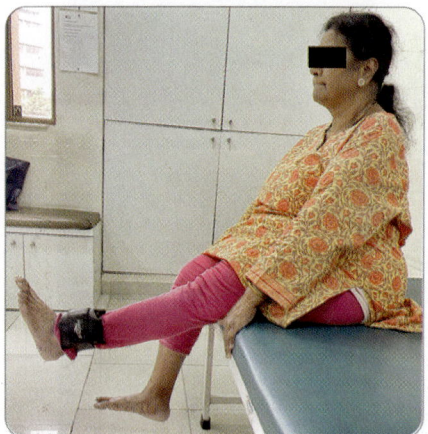 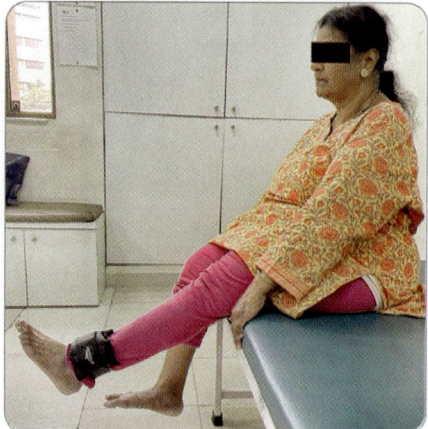

FIG. 14.22: Dynamic quadriceps (90°) with weight cuff.

FIG. 14.23: Dynamic quadriceps (60°) with weight cuff.

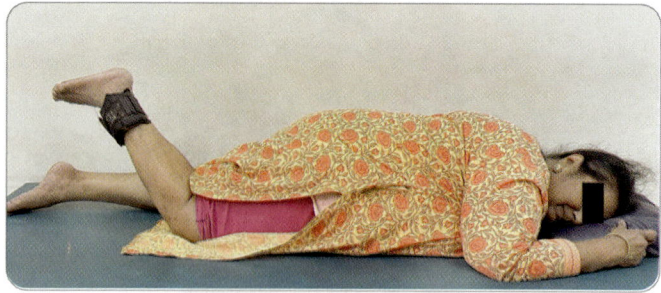

FIG. 14.24: Hamstring curls (with weight cuff).

CHAPTER 14: Rehabilitation in Robotic-guided Knee Arthroplasty

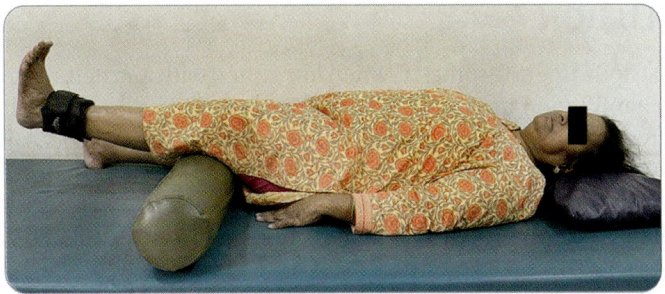

FIG. 14.25: Vastus medialis obliquus (VMO) activation (with weight cuff).

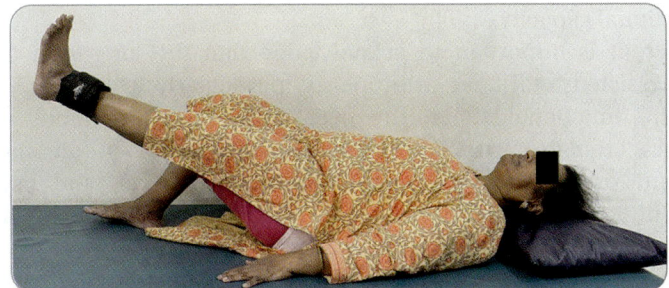

FIG. 14.26: Straight leg raise (SLR) (with weight cuff).

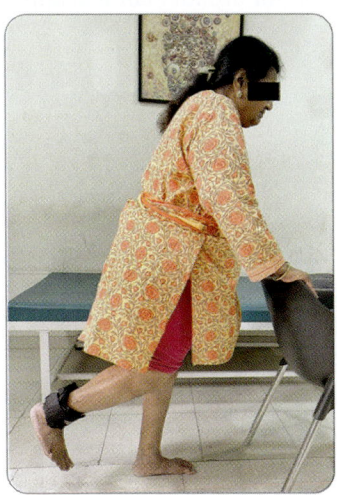

FIG. 14.27: Hip extension (with weight cuff).

CONCLUSION

Robotic-assisted knee arthroplasty, when integrated with a structured and patient-centered rehabilitation approach—including prehabilitation and individualized postoperative therapy—offers a promising pathway to enhance early surgical outcomes. The precision of robotic assistance contributes to improved implant alignment and soft tissue balance, which in turn may lead to better pain control, early mobility, and enhanced functional recovery during the initial postoperative period.

Prehabilitation plays a vital complementary role by optimizing a patient's physical and psychological readiness for surgery. Evidence suggests that patients who undergo targeted preoperative strengthening, education, and conditioning experience reduced postoperative pain, faster return of joint mobility, and overall better functional capacity.

However, it is important to acknowledge that the long-term advantages of robotic-assisted total knee arthroplasty, particularly in terms of prosthetic survivorship, functional superiority over conventional methods, and cost-effectiveness, remain areas of ongoing investigation. Additionally, since each patient presents unique anatomical, physiological, and psychosocial characteristics, rehabilitation protocols must be meticulously tailored to individual goals and limitations to maximize recovery.

In conclusion, the synergy of robotic precision with structured, personalized rehabilitation—starting before surgery and continuing postoperatively—marks a significant advancement in knee arthroplasty care. Thus, high-quality, longitudinal studies are necessary to validate these early benefits and evidence based standardized protocols for broader clinical application.

Suggested Readings

1. Doan GW, Courtis RP, Wyss JG, Green EW, Clary CW. Image-free robotic-assisted total knee arthroplasty improves implant alignment accuracy: A cadaveric study. J Arthroplasty. 2022;37(4):795-801.
2. Murgier J, Clatworthy M. Variable rotation of the femur does not affect outcome with patient specific alignment navigated balanced TKA. Knee Surg Sports Traumatol Arthrosc. 2022;30(2):517-26.
3. An VVG, Twiggs J, Leie M, Fritsch BA. Kinematic alignment is bone and soft tissue preserving compared to mechanical alignment in total knee arthroplasty. Knee 2019;26(2):466-76.
4. Bellemans J, Colyn W, Vandenneucker H, Victor J. The Chitranjan Ranawat award: is neutral mechanical alignment normal for all patients? The concept of constitutional varus. Clin Orthop Relat Res. 2012;470(1):45-53.
5. Hirschmann MT, Karlsson J, Becker R. Hot topic: alignment in total knee arthroplasty-systematic versus more individualised alignment strategies. Knee Surg Sports Traumatol Arthrosc. 2018;26(6):1587-8.
6. Clatworthy M. Outcome & survival analysis of conventional measured resection, neutral alignment Attune TKA vs CAS anatomic tibia, balanced femur, constitutional alignment Attune TKA. Orthop J Sports Med. 2017;5(5_suppl5):2325967117S0015.
7. Marchand RC, Sodhi N, Khlopas A, Sultan AA, Harwin SF, Malkani AL, et al. Patient satisfaction outcomes after robotic arm-assisted total knee arthroplasty: A short-term evaluation. J Knee Surg. 2017;30(9):849-53.
8. Kayani B, Konan S, Tahmassebi J, Pietrzak JRT, Haddad FS. Robotic-arm assisted total knee arthroplasty is associated with improved early functional recovery and reduced time to hospital discharge compared with conventional jig-based total knee arthroplasty: a prospective cohort study. Bone Joint J. 2018;100-B(7):930-7.
9. Agarwal N, To K, McDonnell S, Khan W. Clinical and radiological outcomes in robotic-assisted total knee arthroplasty: A systematic review and meta-analysis. J Arthroplasty. 2020;35(11):3393-409.
10. Vermue H, Lambrechts J, Victor J, Arnout N, Auvinet E, Victor J. How should we evaluate robotics in the operating theatre? Bone Joint J 2020;102-B(4):407-13.
11. Londhe SB, Shetty S, Shetty V, Desouza C, Banka P, Antao N. Comparison of Time Taken in Conventional versus Active Robotic-Assisted Total Knee Arthroplasty. Clin Orthop Surg. 2024;16(2):259-64.
12. Londhe SB, Shetty S, Vora NL, Shah A, Nair R, Shetty V. Evaluation of the safety and efficacy of the fully automated active robotic system in robotic assisted total knee arthroplasty. J Clin Orthop Trauma. 2023;37:102106.
13. Londhe SB, Patel K, Baranwal G. Imageless Robotic Arm-Assisted Total Knee Arthroplasty: Workflow Optimization, Operative Times, and Learning Curve. Cureus. 2025;17(2):e78880.
14. Londhe SB, Patel K, Baranwal GK, Shah A, Shah D. Role of Image-Free Robotic-Assisted Technology in Enhancing Accuracy of Implant Sizing for Total Knee Arthroplasty. Cureus. 2024;16(11):e74256.
15. Londhe SB, Rudraraju RT, Shah R, Desouza C, Shetty VD, Khan FS, et al. Analysis of robot-specific operative time and surgical team anxiety level and its effect on alignment during robot-assisted TKA. J Robot Surg. 2024;18(1):86.
16. Van der List JP, McDonald LS, Pearle AD. Systematic review of medial versus lateral survivorship in uni compartmental knee arthroplasty. Knee Elsevier. 2015;22:454-60.

17. Song EK, Seon JK, Yim JH, Netravali NA, Bargar WL. Robotic-assisted TKA reduces postoperative alignment outliers and improves gap balance compared to conventional TKA knee. Clin Orthop Relat Res. 2013;471:118-26.
18. Moon YW, Ha C, Do KH, Kim CY, Han JH, Na SE, et al. Comparison of robot-assisted and conventional total knee arthroplasty: a controlled cadaver study using multiparameter quantitative three- dimensional CT assessment of alignment. Comput Aided Surg. 2012;17:86-95.
19. Chun YS, Kim KI, Cho YJ, Kim YH, Yoo MC, Rhyu KH. Causes and patterns of aborting a robot-assisted arthroplasty. J Arthroplasty. Elsevier Inc. 2011;26:621-5.
20. Nogalo C, Meena A, Abermann E, Fink C. Complications and downsides of the robotic total knee arthroplasty: a systematic review. Knee Surg Sports Traumatol Arthrosc. 2023;31(3):736-50.
21. Ponzio DY, Lonner JH. Preoperative mapping in unicompartmental knee arthroplasty using computed tomography scans is associated with radiation exposure and carries high cost. J Arthroplasty Elsevier Inc. 2015;30:964-7.
22. Saad A, Mayne A, Pagkalos J, Ollivier M, Botchu R, Davis E, et al. Comparative analysis of radiation exposure in robot-assisted total knee arthroplasty using popular robotic systems. J Robotic Surg. 2024;18:120.
23. Beldame J, Boisrenoult P, Beaufils P. Pin track induced fractures around computer-assisted TKA. Orthop Traumatol Surg Res. 2010;96(3):249-55.
24. Brown MJ, Matthews JR, Bayers-Thering MT, Phillips MJ, Krackow KA. Low incidence of postoperative complications with navigated total knee arthroplasty. J Arthroplasty. 2017;32(7):2120-6.
25. Lang JE, Mannava S, Floyd AJ, Goddard MS, Smith BP, Mofidi A, et al. Robotic systems in orthopaedic surgery. J Bone Joint Surg Br. 2011;93:1296-9.
26. Hohmann E, Bryant A, Tetsworth K. Anterior pelvic soft tissue thickness influences acetabular cup positioning with imageless navigation. J Arthroplast. 2012;27:945-52.
27. Jacofsky DJ, Allen M. Robotics in arthroplasty: a comprehensive review. J Arthroplast. 2016;31:2353-63.
28. Bourne RB, Chesworth BM, Davis AM, Mahomed NN, Charron KD. Patient satisfaction after total knee arthroplasty: Who is satisfied and who is not? Clin Orthop Relat Res. 2010;468:57-63.
29. Gunaratne R, Pratt DN, Banda J, Fick DP, Khan RJK, Robertson BW. Patient Dissatisfaction Following Total Knee Arthroplasty: A Systematic Review of the Literature. J Arthroplasty. 2017;32:3854-60.
30. Abdel MP, Ledford CK, Kobic A, Taunton MJ, Hanssen AD. Contemporary failure aetiologies of the primary, posterior-stabilised total knee arthroplasty. Bone Jt J. 2017;99B:647-52.
31. Marchand RC, Sodhi N, Anis HK, Ehiorobo JO, Mohamed NS, Mont MA. Robotic-arm assisted total knee arthroplasty demonstrated improved accuracy and precision compared with manual technique. J Knee Surg. 2019;32(3):239-50.
32. Lei K, Liu LM, Guo L. Robotic systems in total knee arthroplasty: Current surgical trauma perspectives. Burns Trauma. 2022:10tkac049.
33. Bhor P, Pawar S, Kutumbe D, Vatkar A, Kale S, Jagtap R. Does preoperative 3D CT planning helps in predicting the component size determination and alignment in automatic robotic total knee arthroplasty (RA-TKA). J Orthop. 2023;43:25-9.
34. Plaskos C, Wakelin E, Shalhoub S, Lawrence J, Keggi J, Koenig J, et al. Soft tissue release rate in robot-assisted gap balancing and measurement of cross-sectional total knee arthroplasty. Orthop Proc. 2019;102-B Suppl 2:1.
35. Tang Q, Shang P, Zheng G, Xu HZ, Liu HX. Extramedullary versus intramedullary femoral alignment technique in total knee arthroplasty: A meta-analysis of randomized controlled trials. J Orthop Surg Res. 2017;12:82.
36. Kayani B, Konan S, Tahmassebi J, Pietrzak JRT, Haddad FS. Robotic-arm assisted total knee arthroplasty is associated with improved early functional recovery and reduced time to hospital discharge compared with conventional jig-based total knee arthroplasty: a prospective cohort study. Bone Joint J. 2018;100-B(7):930-7.

37. Raj S, Bola H, York T. Robotic-assisted knee replacement surgery & infection: A historical foundation, systematic review and meta-analysis. J Orthop. 2023;40:38-46.
38. Park CH, Seon JK, Lee KB, Han HS, Lee DH. The impact of robotic-assisted knee arthroplasty on early functional recovery and complications: a multicenter study. J Orthop Surg Res. 2022;17(1):135.
39. Alrayes MM, Sukeik M. Robotics in total knee replacement: Current use and future implications. World J Orthop. 2024;15(6):489-94.
40. Walgrave S, Oussedik S. Comparative assessment of current robotic-assisted systems in primary total knee arthroplasty. Bone Jt Open. 2023;4(1):13-8.
41. Saber AY, Marappa-Ganeshan R, Mabrouk A. Robotic-Assisted Total Knee Arthroplasty. In: StatPearls. Treasure Island (FL): StatPearls Publishing; 2025.
42. Scaturro D, Vitagliani F, Caracappa D, Tomasello S, Chiaramonte R, Vecchio M, et al. Rehabilitation approach in robot assisted total knee arthroplasty: an observational study. BMC Musculoskelet Disord. 2023;24(1):140.
43. Riga M, Altsitzioglou P, Saranteas T, Mavrogenis AF. Enhanced recovery after surgery (ERAS) protocols for total joint replacement surgery. SICOT J. 2023;9:E1.
44. Bhor P, Pawar SH, Kutumbe D, Vatkar AJ, Kale S, Jagtap R. An observational study on the functional outcomes of 100 robotic total knee replacements performed by an Indian surgeon: Early experiences. MGM J Med Sci. 2024;11(1):24-30.
45. Dutta S, Ambade R, Wankhade D, Agrawal P. Rehabilitation Techniques Before and After Total Knee Arthroplasty for a Better Quality of Life. Cureus. 2024;16(2):e54877.

Author's Publications

1. Bhor P, Pawar S, Kutumbe D, Vatkar A, Kale S, Jagtap R. Is Native Joint Line More Accurately Restored with Robotic Assisted Total Knee Arthroplasty than with Conventional Instruments? J Orthop Case Rep. 2025;15(2):233-8.
   Available from https://jocr.co.in/wp/2025/02/01/is-native-joint-line-more-accurately-restored-with-robotic-assisted-total-knee-arthroplasty-than-with-conventional-instruments

2. Bhor P, Pawar SH, Kutumbe D, Vatkar A, Kale S. Robotic-assisted total knee replacement in a patient with severe varus deformity and high cardiac risk: A case report. J Clin Orthop. 2024;9(2):129-31.
   Available from https://jcorth.com/2024/12/10/robotic-assisted-total-knee-replacement-in-a-patient-with-severe-varus-deformity-and-high-cardiac-risk/

3. Bhor P, Pawar S, Ali S, Vatkar A, Kale S, Kutumbe D. The role of computed tomography in achieving true external rotation in robotic knee replacement: A retrospective analysis of 300 knees. J Orthop Case Rep. 2025;15(2):269-74.
   Available from https://jocr.co.in/wp/2025/02/01/the-role-of-computed-tomography-in-achieving-true-external-rotation-in-robotic-knee-replacement-a-retrospective-analysis-of-300-knees

4. Bhor P, Pawar S, Kutumbe D, Vatkar A, Kale S, Jagtap R. An observational study on the functional outcomes of 100 robotic total knee replacements performed by an Indian surgeon: Early experiences. MGM J Med Sci. 2024;11(1):24-30.
   Available from: https://www.researchgate.net/publication/379456766

5. Bhor P, Pawar S, Kutumbe D, Vatkar A, Kale S, Jagtap R. Does preoperative 3D CT planning helps in predicting the component size determination and alignment in automatic robotic total knee arthroplasty (RA-TKA). J Orthop. 2023;43:25-9.
   Available from: https://www.researchgate.net/publication/372586333

Index

Page numbers followed by *f* refer to figure and *t* refer to table.

A

ACCUBALANCE graph 98*f*, 112, 113*f*
  recording 112
Accurate component alignment 173
Active dynamic quadriceps sets 188
Active robotic arm 30
Adaptive planning 87
Advanced navigation 48
Alignment philosophies, evolution in 4
Anatomical alignment 13, 14*f*, 21
  technique strives 13
Anatomical landmark digitalization 154, 157*f*
Angular movements 25
Ankle
  center 57
  pumps 193
  toe
    movement 189, 196
    pumps 197*f*
Anterior chamfer 48, 113
Anterior cortex 109
  anatomic landmark digitization of 159*f*
  registration 111*f*
Anterior femur resection 113
Anteroposterior cut guide 135*f*
Anti-inflammatory food 187
Apex distal 19, 20
Apex proximal 19, 20
Aquatic therapy 196
Arithmetic hip-knee-ankle angle 19, 19*f*
Arm
  calibration attachments 69*f*
  reference frame 144*f*
Array drill pin 94, 95*f*
  placement 99, 101
Array set 93, 94*f*
Array stabilizer 75, 76
Arthritic knee preimplantation 83*f*
Arthroplasty 8*t*
  Robotic system in 32
Arthroscopy 65
Arthrotomy 77, 125
Artificial intelligence, recent advent of 4
ATRACSYS Advanced Tracking System 119
Auto segmentation 38
Autoclavability 61
Automated soft tissue balance 175
Autonomous system, early 9
Axial view 60*f*
Axis point 103

B

Balance training 188, 196
Balanced extension 46
Balanced flexion 46
Balanced soft tissues 183
Base reference frame 145*f*
Base station touchscreen display 91, 91*f*
Baseplate type 74
Bilateral knee replacement 116
Bilateral lower limb scanogram
  preoperative 170*f*
Blood loss 183, 184
Bone
  appropriate depth of 136
  array 102
  conservation 183
  cuts, robotic-assisted 160, 161*f*, 165*f*
  cutting 64, 65*f*, 133
  mapping 84
    registration of 78
    verifications of 78

Index

markers, resection of 114*f*
  pin 76
    insertion of 75, 76
    preparation 75
    registration, status of 70
    removal 134, 136*f*
  resection
    guidance 160, 161*f*
    techniques 175
  saw model 122*f*
  verification of 77
Bony landmark 103*t*
  acquisition 98
Bony preparation 80
Bosu ball, balancing on 191*f*
Breathing exercises 188
Burr systems 27, 28*f*

C

Calcium 187
Calf stretch 187
Calibration errors 181
Camera 36*f*, 141
  adjustment 102
  orientation 126*f*
  position 102*f*
  positioning arm 141
  specifications 72
  vision 54*f*
Cardiovascular fitness training 189
Chest physiotherapy 188
Clinical deformities 79
Close chain exercises 189, 196
Closed platform system 30, 31
Combined lower limb coronal orientation 16
Compact design 138
Components positioning 12, 14, 15
Computed tomography
  free technology 87
  scan 37, 55, 71, 80*f*
    positioning for 56*f*
    rod for 56*f*
    tips for 71
Condyle center 57
Constitutional limb alignment 19, 21

Conventional total knee replacement 1, 115
Cooling system 27
Core strengthening exercises 188, 193
CORI console 118, 119*f*
  power rating 118
CORI robotic system 118
CORI software 124
CORI system, proper setup of 124
CORI-assisted surgery 125
Coronal knee alignment 20
Coronal limb alignment, adjustment of 16
Coronal plane alignment of knee 21
  applicability of 21
  classification 20*f*
  strength of 21
Coronal section
  medial-lateral fit 59
  mesiolingual fit 60*f*
Cryotherapy 193, 194, 196
Cutter blade specifications 73
Cutting system 55*f*, 143
Cutting tool 23, 31, 54
  and chuck system 54
  sleeve 54
Cutting-edge solution 29
CUVIS joint robotic system 33
CUVIS preplanner software 35
CUVIS robotic system 9, 37*f*
  components of 33, 34*f*

D

Debris management, irrigation sleeve for 54
Deep vein thrombosis 189
Diaphragmatic breathing 188
Diet 187
Digital tensiometer 132*f*
Digital tensioner 131
Distal condyles digitizer 146
Distal directions 78
Distal femoral
  condyle 107
    registration 110*f*
  cutting jig, placement of 161*f*

Distal femur 62
    resection 113
Distal precision burring 121
Distal resection 135*f*
Drill guide 125
Dynamic kinematic assessment 154, 160*f*
Dynamic quadriceps 198*f*

Elliptical training 189
Enhanced recovery after surgery 186
Enhanced tibial slope accuracy 173
Ergonomic handpiece 118, 119*f*
Erroneous soft tissue balancing 176
Exaggerated femoral bow 2*f*
Extendable robotic arm 69
External femoral reference placement 152*f*

F

Fatigue reduction 184
Femoral anatomy, data of 25
Femoral array 68*f*
Femoral axis 56
Femoral center acquisition 103, 104*f*
Femoral checkpoints position 78*f*
Femoral condyles 84
Femoral cuts 162*f*
Femoral implant planning screen 59*f*
Femoral joint line obliquity 15
Femoral marker, movement of 25
Femoral mechanical-anatomical axis angle 1
Femoral pin 45*f*
    insertion, position of 76*f*
Femoral reference
    frame 147*f*
    placement
        inside incision 151, 152*f*
        outside incision 151
Femoral registration 57
    points 58*f*
Femoral resections 18
Femur 77, 81*f*, 101, 125, 131, 136*f*
    anterior chamfer cut 80

array placement in 101*f*
axis 38
bone removal 135*f*
checkpoint 78, 99, 100*f*
cut guide for 122*f*
distal cut 82
free collection 128*f*
implant
    fit 131
    position 39, 39*f*
knee center 107, 108*f*
pin placement 101*f*
points collection on 44*f*
posterior chamfer cut 82
postresection of 48*f*
puresight hydrophobic optical markers of 90*f*
registration points 40
resection of 115
tracker 120*f*
Final bone
    mapping 63, 63*f*
    resection 161*f*
Final distal femoral bone cut 162*f*
Final implant placement 166
Final leg assessment 114, 114*f*
Final root mean square 42
First robot-assisted human hip replacement 9
Flat markers 24
Flexible imaging options 148
Foot pedal 119
Footprint size 70
Forward-backward waking 194
Freedom
    degrees of 70
    knee 41
Functional alignment 17, 18*f*

Gait training 188
Gap assessment 132*f*
Gap balancing 63, 64*f*, 84
    technique of 46*t*
Gap planning 132
Geometric configuration 25

Glass
  lens marker 24
  marker 25f

H

Hamstring 188
  curls 198f
  matrix therapy for 189f
  stretch 187, 190f
Haptic feedback 27
  sensors 27
Haptics-using robotic arm interactive orthopedic system 66
Head center 57
Heel-to-toe walking 188
Higher knee society scores 174
Higher satisfaction scores 173
High-speed
  burr 138
  cutting motor 54
Hip
  abduction 191f, 193, 198f
  center 158f
    registration 127f
    verification screen 77f
  extension 199f
    strengthening 195
  flexors stretch 187
  joint, reduce medial and lateral motion of 84
  knee-ankle 30, 141, 166
  mobility exercises 193
  strengthening 193
Huffing-coughing 188
Humanoid footprint 52f
Hybrid alignment 17
Hydration 187

I

Image-based processing systems, types of 30, 181
Image-free real-time mapping 138
Imageless systems 30, 31
Implant
  insertion 48
  misalignment 176
  planning 58, 79, 129, 132
  positioning 17
  trialing 137
Incentive spirometry 188
Infection 176
Infrared light, principle of 23
Initial bone mapping 62, 62f
Initial leg alignment 112
Initial proadjust surgical planning 112
Insert femoral pins 76
Interactive device 23, 27, 142
Interactive screen 28f
Intramedullary canal 1
Intramedullary femoral rodding 179f
Intramedullary rod, wobble of 2f
Intraoperative anatomical mapping 148
Intraoperative bone surface marking 79f
Intraoperative planning 74, 75
Intraoperative protocols 62
Intraoperative registration 154
Intraoperative scenario 46, 81f
Inverse kinematic alignment 18, 18f
  principle of 140

J

Joint
  balancing 75, 79
  kinematics 172
  line
    inclination 13-15
    obliquity 19, 20f
    orientation angle 13, 15

K

Kinematic alignment 15, 15f, 16f, 21
  principle of 15, 44
  proponents of 16
Knee 93
  arthroplasty 177
    real intelligence CORI for 119
    robotic-assisted 185, 200
  classification, coronal plane alignment of 19
  continuous passive movement for 193
  coronal plane alignment of 20, 21
  femoral array 77

Index

final 3D model of 42*f*
joint 6, 79
  exposure 42
  natural deformities of 74
osteoarthritis 185
postoperative X-ray of 170*f*
preoperative X-ray of 170*f*
region 71
replacement 84
  modern 6
  revision surgery 176
  surgery 6
  unicompartmental 175
tibia validation tool 147*f*

L

Laminar spreader 131
Lateral condyle center 57
Lateral distal condyle 57
  anatomic landmark digitization of 159*f*
Lateral distal femoral angle 19, 20
Lateral epicondyle 57, 84
Lateral plateau points 106*f*
Lateral posterior condyle 57
Learning curve 172, 175
Leg
  passive movements of 158*f*
  positioner 77
    kit 75*f*
  positioning 84
Ligament
  balance
    gaps 115*f*
    graph 98*f*
  balancing, errors in 3
Ligamental tensioning 81*f*
Limb
  alignment assessment 75
  flexion of 127*f*
Low-intensity class III laser 189*f*

M

Machine learning integration 175
Mako cutting system 72
Mako display system 78
MAKO navigation system 74*f*
MAKO robotic arm 74*f*
  assisted system 66
MAKO robotic system 9, 24, 30, 66, 67*f*
Mako saw blade 73*f*
Mako system empowers surgeons 85
Mako tips and tricks 83
Mako total knee arthroplasty
  software application, planning methodology of 73
  system 66
Malalignment-related revision rates 174
Malunited fractures 2, 3*f*
Matrix
  size 55
  therapy 189*f*
Mechanical alignment 13*f*, 14, 16, 21, 141
  gold standard of 12
Mechanical deformities 79
Medial condyle center 57
Medial distal condyle 57
  anatomic landmark digitization of 158*f*
Medial epicondyle 57, 84
Medial malleolus 77
Medial plateau points 106*f*
Medial posterior condyle 57
Medial proximal tibial angle 20
Medical field, robotic in 8
Meril implant, posterior condylar cut values for 59
Metal rod 36
Minimal pain around knee 193
Minimally invasive robotic knee arthroplasty 186, 193
  postoperative rehabilitation protocol for 193*t*
  preoperative rehabilitation protocol for 186*t*
Minimized soft tissue damage 183
MISSO design specifications 52*t*
MISSO pre-planner software 55
MISSO robot cart 52
MISSO robotic
  arm 52
  software 55
  system 10, 51, 51*f*
MISSO vision cart 52

Mobility 193-195
Multi-angle vastus medialis obliquus
    activation 195
Multicenter analysis 174
Multiplane array system 72
Multiple angle quadriceps strengthening 195
Muscle memory, low threshold
    strengthening exercises for 188
Myofascial release 196

N

Natural knee 13
    alignment 14
    kinematics 174
Navigation screen 79*f*
Navigation tracker visibility 154
    confirmation of 156*f*
NAVIO robotic system 9
Network device interface 52
    camera 53*f*
    optical camera 24*f*
Neuromuscular electrical stimulation
    189, 193, 196
Neurosurgery 8
Nonimage-based navigation, principles
    of 140
Nutrition 187

O

Open chain exercises 188, 189, 196
Open platform system 30
Operating room 34
    setup in 125*f*
    space in 87
    system layout in 47*f*
Operation theater setup 64*f*
Optical camera 23, 141
Optical tracker 72, 142
    hygiene 84
Optical tracking system 23, 33, 53, 141
    components of 143*f*
Optical unit 141
Optimal alignment 166
Optimal camera position 155*f*

Orthopedic
    robotic in 8
    surgery 29, 177
Osteoarthritic knees 21
Osteophytes 44
    exposure of 98
    incision of 98
    removal of 98

P

Pain management 187
Passive robotic arm 30
Passive system 31
Patellar mobilization 194, 195, 197*f*
Patient landmark 74
    registration 84
Periarticular femoral pin placement 179*f*
Perturbation training 188
Phenotype classification 20
Pin 25
    placement 43*f*, 62*f*, 83, 115, 125
Planar articulation 93
Planning device 33
Point probe 123, 123*f*
Polyethylene 168*f*
Postbony resection gap balancing 82
Post-condylar bone resection 41
Posterior chamfer 48, 113
Posterior condylar
    anatomic landmark digitization of 158*f*
    bone resection values 61*t*
    cuts 41*f*
    digitizer 146, 146*f*
Posterior cruciate ligament
    anatomic landmark digitization of 160*f*
    fossa center 57
Posterior femoral condyles 109
    registration 111*f*
Posterior femur resection 113
Posterior stabilized knee surgery 113
Postoperative gap assessment 137*f*
Postoperative pain
    minimized 173
    reduced 174
Postresection extension gap check 49*f*
Postresection flexion gap check 49*f*

Post-trial implant ligamental balancing 82*f*
Precise bone cuts 174
Pre-resection extension gap check 45*f*
Pre-resection flexion gap check 45*f*
Pre-resection joint tensioning 80
Proadjust surgical planning 102, 113*f*
Probe tracker frame 26*f*
Procut saw blade 94, 95*f*
Proprioception training 188
Proximal center 57
Proximal directions 78
Proximal tibia 168*f*
Proximal tibial
   cut 80, 166*f*
   cutting jig, placement of 165*f*
   resection 113
Pulmonary embolism 184

Q

Quadriceps
   activation 195
   isometric exercise for 188
   matrix therapy for 189*f*
   muscle, matrix rhythm therapy for 194, 196
   stretch 187, 190*f*
Quicker rehabilitation 173

R

Radiation exposure 177
Range of motion 127*f*
   active 196
   passive 196
   training 187
Rasp 123, 123*f*
Real-time adjustments 170
Real-time data system 87
Real-time kinematic assessment 149
Recurvatum 79
Reflective markers 24
Registration
   malfunctions 180
   pointer 145*f*

Rehabilitation
   goals of 186-189, 193-196
   minimally invasive robotic knee arthroplasty 186-189, 193-196
   phases of 186-189, 193-196
   postoperative protocol 193
Repeat landmark acquisition 111, 112*f*
Restricted kinematic alignment 141
Rigid body tools 25
Robot 8
   arm 23, 26, 29, 31, 33, 34, 35*f*, 47*f*, 67*f*
   dimensions 52, 87, 88*t*
   over-reliance 84
   placement 63, 64*f*, 83
   preparation 61
   weight 88*t*
Robotic 1
   device, status indicator on 93
   dimensions 118*t*
   distal cut guide 121
   evolution of 6
   guidance 143
   history of 6
   Mako knee replacement surgery 85
   surgery 8*t*, 26*f*, 30, 32, 54*f*
   weight 118*t*
Robotic arm
   base array 68*f*
   calibration 70
   control 71
   cutting process 31
   functionality of 30
   mills 48
   specifications 52, 70, 141
   with six axes 27*f*
Robotic cart 118
   power rating 118
Robotic drill 120, 121*f*
   and burs 120
Robotic system
   classification of 30
   components of 23
   image of 67
   modern 29
Robotic total knee replacement 115
   advantages of 182

Index

Robotic-assisted device 92, 93f
Robotic-assisted surgery 85, 182
　advent of 140
Robotic-assisted system 4
Robotic-assisted technologies 4
Robotic-guided pin-hole placement 163f, 164f
ROSA accuracy, key benefits of 172
ROSA arm reference frame 144, 144f
ROSA knee
　condyle digitizer 146
　system 9, 141f, 150f, 172
　　dimensions 142f
　　instrumentation 144
　　working radius of 143f
　tibia validation tool 146
ROSA nonimage-based robotic total knee replacement
　accuracy and precision in 171
　benefits over traditional techniques in 172
　challenges and future perspectives of 174
　clinical outcomes of 173
　surgical workflow of 149
ROSA registration 157f
　pointer 145
ROSA robotic system 140
ROSA system 151f, 163f, 166f, 167f, 169f
ROSA total knee arthroplasty cut guide 145
ROSA workflow, advantages of 170
Rossum's universal robots 8
Rotation alignment 164f

S

Satellite station 92f, 92t
　specifications 91
　touchscreen 91
　transfer mechanism 92
Saw blades 121
Saw system 27, 28f, 65
Segmental expansion exercise 188
Self-retraction system 77
Semiactive robotic arm 30
Shock wave 187
Short oblique periprosthetic femoral fracture 179f
Shorter learning curve 173
Single-leg
　clock taps 188
　stance 188, 191f
Sit-to-stand transfer training 193
Six-axis design 53f
Soft tissue
　balancing 166, 171, 172, 174
　injuries 180
　manipulation 193
　mobilization around knee joint 194, 195
　release 16, 187
Software glitches 181
Spherical marker 24f
Stair climbing practice 188
Standard surgical tool 143
Static cycling 189, 194, 196
Static quadriceps 190f, 193
Sterile drapes 95
Sterilization 61
　method of 95
Straight leg raise 189, 191f, 196, 199f
Stryker Mako optical tracking system
　details 72
Stryker Mako robotic system
　specifications 69
Stryker Mako total knee arthroplasty
　surgical steps 75
Superior-inferior glide 195
Surgery
　robotic-assisted 85, 182
　selection 74
Surgical planning 37
　process of 38f
　protocol 124
Swelling around knee 193
System initialization 154

T

Tandem
　stance 188
　walking 188
Theraband 195

Thoracic expansion 188
Tibia 40, 77, 81*f*, 125, 131, 136*f*
  array placement in 101*f*
  axis 40, 130*f*
  bone removal 135*f*
  checkpoint 78
  coronal alignment 80
  cut guide selection 134*f*
  free collection 129*f*
  implant positioning 40
  malleoli of 160*f*
  pin insertion, position of 76*f*
  points collection on 44*f*
  points for 62
  postresection of 48*f*
  puresight hydrophobic optical markers of 90*f*
  resection of 115
  tracker 120*f*
  twin peg for 121
Tibial array 68*f*
Tibial axis 56
Tibial checkpoint 99, 99*f*
  position 78*f*
Tibial component placement 168*f*
Tibial implant positioning 40*f*, 131
Tibial knee center 105, 105*f*
Tibial mechanical axis 56, 103, 104*f*, 105*f*
Tibial pin placement 100*f*
Tibial plateau 106, 160*f*
Tibial posterior slope 46
Tibial reference
  frames 146, 147*f*
  placement
    inside incision 154*f*
    outside incision 153, 153*f*
Tibial registration 58
  points 40, 59*f*
Tibial resection level 106*f*
Tibial sagittal axis 107, 107*f*
Tibial slope 108*f*
Tibial tracking arrays 134
Total hip arthroplasty 9
Total knee arthroplasty 3, 6, 7, 72, 182
  alignment strategies in 12
  anatomic alignment for 13
  cut guide 145*f*
  lateral X-ray of 179*f*
  preoperative rehabilitation for 186
  robotic-assisted 66, 177
Total knee replacement 1, 4, 86, 140, 182
  procedure of 37*f*
  robotic-assisted revision 175
Touch interface 70
Touchscreen
  medical-grade monitor 53
  tablet 119
Tracker
  balls 24
  frames 25
  placement 151
Tracking system 36*f*
Transepicondylar axis 13, 14, 38, 164*f*
  angle 39*f*
Transversus abdominis 189, 196
Treadmill walking 189, 192*f*
Trial implants 166
Troccaz classification 31, 32*f*
Tuberosity 57
Twin peg cut guide 136*f*

U

Universal validation tool body 145
Unstable joint 176
Upper body ergometer 189

V

Valgus
  deformity 79
  limb alignment 20
Validation tool body 146*f*
Varus
  deformity cut 61
  valgus 25
Vastus medialis obliquus 196
  activation 199*f*
VELYS base station 88
  console 90, 91*f*
  footswitch 90, 91*f*
  touchscreen 90
VELYS camera 89, 89*f*
VELYS graphical user interface 96

VELYS ligament sensor tensor 95, 96*f*
VELYS reusable instruments 95, 96*f*
VELYS robotic assisted device 92, 93
VELYS robotic assisted solutions 10, 86
   key features of 87
VELYS robotic assisted system
   advantages 115
   disadvantages 116
VELYS robotic system 86, 87*f*, 88
   main components of 88*f*
VELYS satellite station 88
VELYS screen 97*f*
VELYS single use instruments 93
VELYS system, setting up 97
Virtual planning 160
Vision system 35, 36*f*, 52, 119
   markers of 36*f*, 43*f*

Visualizing bone removal 136*f*
Vitamin D 187

W

Weight 52, 69, 195
   bearing 197*f*
   cuff 191*f*, 198*f*, 199*f*
   management 187
   shifting 188
      exercises 188
Whiteside's line 107, 109*f*
Working radius 70, 141

Z

Zig-zag walking 194
Z-retractor 131